I0023216

James Clark

The Ladies' Guide to Beauty

James Clark

The Ladies' Guide to Beauty

ISBN/EAN: 9783337225728

Printed in Europe, USA, Canada, Australia, Japan

Cover: Foto ©Lupo / pixelio.de

More available books at **www.hansebooks.com**

THE

LADIES' GUIDE TO BEAUTY

CONTAINING

PRACTICAL ADVICE ON IMPROVING THE COMPLEXION, THE
HAIR, THE HANDS, THE FORM, THE TEETH, THE EYES,
THE FEET, THE FEATURES; SO AS TO INSURE THE
HIGHEST DEGREE OF PERFECTION OF WHICH
THEY ARE SUSCEPTIBLE.

AND ALSO,

UPWARDS OF ONE HUNDRED RECIPES FOR VARIOUS
COSMETICS, OILS, POMADES, ETC. ETC.,

BEING THE RESULT OF A COMBINATION OF

PRACTICAL AND SCIENTIFIC SKILL.

BY SIR JAMES CLARK,

PRIVATE PHYSICIAN TO QUEEN VICTORIA.

REVISED AND EDITED BY AN AMERICAN PHYSICIAN AND CHEMIST.

NEW YORK:

DICK & FITZGERALD, PUBLISHERS,

18 ANN STREET.

INTRODUCTION.

FEMALE BEAUTY! this is our subject; this the object we shall show how to obtain; and if we can assist nature in perfecting her most glorious work, or enable her to preserve it in perfection for years after her unassisted efforts would have failed, our names will be registered among those of the greatest benefactors of mankind; for are not all alive to its influence, all slaves to its power? For it the muse has exerted its happiest efforts; warriors and statesmen have arisen by its inspiration; for it Petrarch wasted a life,* and Marc Antony lost a world.

In prosecuting our object we shall occasionally be compelled to introduce certain cosmetics to the notice of our readers; in so doing we shall constantly bear in mind that many preparations which temporarily improve the appearance of the skin, will ultimately, not only destroy its beauty, but injure the general health; we shall carefully exclude all such from our pages; no deleterious compound shall be employed under our

---

* "For twenty years of his life love was the main-spring of his actions, and he was perpetually travelling. When at Avignon or Vaucluse he wished to be transported to his beloved Italy; and when in Italy, he could only think of the shades and solitudes of Vaucluse, frequently flying from Avignon to banish, if possible, the remembrance of his Laura, and as often plunging into the solitudes of Vaucluse to avoid her disdain."—*Biography of Petrarch.*

sanction. Health is the fountain of beauty, and we
shall, *en passant*, give such sanative admonitions as will
tend to confirm it in the robust, and to impart it to the
debilitated—without, however, usurping the province of
the family physician, or exposing ourselves to the charge
of that recklessness which characterizes the quack-doctor.

Independent of the serious injury to health which is
frequently caused by the use of compositions, of the
chemical qualities of which the persons who use them
have no idea, much inconvenience arises from their producing effects the direct opposite of that intended—
against such we shall guard our fair readers, by inform-
ing them that they are generally made of oxides of
bismuth, or of lead, which are peculiarly susceptible of
atmospheric influence; and whenever these come in contact with sulphuretted hydrogen, the face of the wearer
will immediately become black.

Our readers will probably have heard a story (fre
quently related by chemical lecturers) which ludicrously
illustrates the danger of using cosmetics, which are
vended as regenerators of beauty, without some better
recommendation than the assurance of the persons most
interested in the disposal of the nostrum. Lest, however, any should not have heard it, we shall repeat tho
oft-told tale.

"A lady who had been in the habit of using a face
powder, commonly called pearl white, (the white oxide
of bismuth,) attended a lecture, during which many
chemical experiments were exhibited; among others,
various medicated waters were analyzed, and occasionally these waters were handed to the company for their
examination; the Harrowgate waters, which are strongly
impregnated with sulphuretted hydrogen, coming under

the notice of the lecturer, he directed the attention of
the lady to its peculiar effluvia, and the moment it was
advanced towards the face of the ' fair unconscious,' that
very fair face became perfectly black, to the great hor-
ror of the majority of the audience, who, being ignorant
of the cause of the change, imagined that she had been
suddenly seized with some frightful malady : their fears,
however, were quieted when the lecturer perceived the
accident, and explained the chemical combination which
had taken place; the lady was, of course, exceedingly
annoyed by being made such a fright, and doubtless not
a little vexed at the publicity given to the fact that all
her charms were not derived from nature." Any of our
readers may be subjected to similar mortification by the
use of a cosmetic in which the white oxide of bismuth
is introduced; the atmosphere is, in some cases, sufficiently impregnated with such exhalations as will affect
the bismuth ; the railway engine frequently gives out sufficient sulphuretted hydrogen when passing through a tun-
nel, to ensure a complete discoloration of a face upon
which pearl white had been powdered ; we cannot therefore too seriously impress upon our fair friends the necessity of care in using drugs which are advertised as
assistants to, or regenerators of, beauty.

In adopting our advice they may rely wherever we
recommend a cosmetic, that it will be wholly free from
anything deleterious.

THE

LADIES' GUIDE TO BEAUTY.

CHAPTER I.

BEAUTY OF FORM.

INFANCY—MEDICAL HINTS TO MOTHERS, TO AID THEM IN SECURING THE
HEALTH AND IN IMPROVING THE BEAUTY OF THEIR OFFSPRING. BAND-
AGES FREQUENTLY THE CAUSE OF DEFORMITIES AND SPINAL AFFEC-
TIONS.

BEFORE we introduce our readers to the various modes of
preserving the beauty which nature has imparted and of remedying defects which have, from whatsoever cause, arisen,
i. e., when they can be remedied or concealed, we must say a
few words to Mothers, as the foundation of personal beauty
must be laid in infancy. To our Mothers and Nurses we must
be indebted for perfection of form ; if any injury arises from
the negligence of either, in after life it will be too late to attempt an absolute remedy to the distortions produced in infancy ; the injured spine or shoulder can only be hidden ; the
weakened joints can only be assisted ; the deformed leg can
scarcely be concealed ; we shall therefore recommend such at-
tentions and practices as with ordinary care will secure to the
infant all the advantages which nature conferred, and repair
many defects which nature, or the habits of the mother previous to the birth of her infant, may have imparted ; and when
the infant has risen into childhood, the mother will find in our
little tome directions for a physical and moral training, which
(except in cases of chronic disorder) shall secure health to her
offspring, " that great fountain of personal beauty."

If the mother, then, wishes to secure health and beauty for her child, her precautions must commence ere its birth; for she must resolve to abandon that absurd system of tight lacing of the stays, which is now so common, and, under any circumstances, is so injurious, but especially so during pregnancy: in the second chapter we have gone into this subject at large, therefore we shall here only point out the evils which may arise from the practice during pregnancy. This unnatural pressure produces very numerous malformations of the infant, among others, twisted ankles or feet—club feet—and inferior development of the various organs and limbs, and it is not to be doubted that the mental powers of the future infant may be affected by the unnatural pressure imposed upon the *fœtus.* Mrs. Walker has some sensible remarks upon this subject, which we quote for the benefit of our readers: " Women in a state of pregnancy should wear nothing that can exercise the slightest compression on any *one* part of the body.

" If constriction of the chest disposes females to irritation of the lungs, and leads to phthisis, &c., this effect will be much more rapidly produced during pregnancy, when the organs of the abdomen being pressed against the lungs, diminish the expansion of the upper cavity, and produce difficulty of respiration. The pressure of clothing over the chest produces either inflammatory swellings or wasting away of the breast. It produces also imperfect secretion of milk, with all the inconveniences that thence result, both to the mother and child. It may give rise to fatal hemorrhages and apoplexy. Pressure of the clothes upon the abdomen, is not less pernicious; it either forces the inferior organs to follow in their development a vertical direction, and leads to all the accidents of which we have spoken, or opposes the development and growth of the infant, and may even cause abortion."

Having thus guarded the mother upon the subject of injuring her child before its birth, we proceed to give a few hints which will aid her in securing to her children health, and its usual accompaniment—beauty.

1.—We will observe, that the personal attention of the mother is one great means of promoting the above object. The natural diet of the child flows from its mother's breast, and no substitute can be so productive of health; if circumstances render it absolutely necessary for the mother to provide a person to perform the truly maternal duty of lactation to, and the bringing up of her infant, let her, by strict attention, see that the duty is properly performed by her substitute.

2.—After having provided for the food of her child, let her

next attention be directed to its being properly washer dressed, and exercised ; let her recollect that in the clothing, ease and warmth are the two all-important points to attend to ; ease can only be obtained by avoiding all unnecessary bandages, which prevent the free use of the joints, and *retard the circulation of the blood*. An infant has been likened to a mass of compressible vessels, through which a fluid is to pass without its circulation being impeded ; these vessels being surrounded by a substance which would not bear any considerable pressure without injury. Keeping this idea in view, how irrational does it appear, that, under the pretence of support, the babe is frequently so tightly bound as to give it continual pain : how should it be other than painful ? A delicate being who an hour before swam in a fluid, to prevent its being injured by the surrounding parts of its mother, bandaged to all but suffocation ! It is monstrous ! When thus absurdly bound, the efforts of an infant to free itself is a common cause of deformity.

3.—See that the infant is carried in a proper position, for on this the future beauty of its form very much depends. For the first two months it should be reclined horizontally ; indeed, this position should be preserved until it shows a desire to sit up ; then, the back and the head should be carefully supported. "*Our* ordinary system of nursing," says a popular writer, " should be termed the art of deforming and weakening children by ill-directed care." And when we consider that very young infants are continually carried in an upright position, it may be properly termed so ; this position is exceedingly painful, and makes the child irritable and fretful ; the bones of the back and neck being separated by a soft gristle, this must be painfully compressed if the weight of the head and body be thrown upon it, before it acquires sufficient firmness ; this habit is also a fruitful source of spinal affections, humpback, and a variety of other deformities. When the child does sit up, take care that the nurse does *not* always carry it upon the same arm.

4.—As the infant advances in age, see that it is carried straight ; that its limbs are properly manipulated ; and if the child cries during the operation, try it yourself, for a lazy nurse may do it too roughly, with a view of making the child dislike that, which should impart pleasure as well as health. Plenty of exercise, plenty of water, and plenty of friction upon the skin, are sources of health from infancy to maturity ; and nothing is more calculated to retard the approaches of age, than habitually laving of the whole body, succeeded by fric tion ; it also beautifies the skin much better than the mos powerful cosmetics, without the disadvantage to which most ot these are subject ; viz., the ultimate injury to the texture of the skin, which all unnatural appliances must produce. These we shall notice under their proper head.

5.—Pay most particular attention to the cleanliness of your infant ; inattention to this lays the foundation of many weaknesses and deformities. Wet under-clothes are vitally injurious. Avoid all swinging cots and cradles ; disease of the brain and squinting are often produced by these apologies for idleness ; the child will, however, never require to be rocked to sleep if proper means be adopted from the time of its birth ; and in no time of life has habit more influence than in infancy.

6.—"Give infants plenty of sleep, milk, and flannel," says Dr. Hunter. At night the child should invariably sleep with its mother, (or her substitute, if she cannot nurse it,) for it has not power to generate sufficient heat, in cold weather especially, even if it be encased in flannel ; the mother's bosom must impart this. There is no danger in the practice of the infant sleeping by its mother's side, as even in sleep she will soon become so accustomed to the presence of her child as to be sensible of its slightest movement. Dr. Ryan estimates that one half of the human race perishes from cold before it arrives at three years of age. Sleep and warmth are essentials to an infant. A child properly clothed and in good health need not fear exposure to the open air even in January : recollect, however, that the clothing of children should be warm, but not heavy.

7.—If you wish your child to retain health, "the fountain of beauty," do not allow narcotics of any description to be administered, but by the advice of your medical man ; and be most jealously on the alert to prevent their clandestine introduction to your nursery. Idle nurses will give them to the infant to render personal attention unnecessary. Narcotics frequently impart a sallowness to the complexion that can never be eradicated, and always injure, if they do not destroy, the constitution, thus retarding the development of the child's form, and even more often producing weakness which prove destructive to incipient beauty.

8.—EXERCISE OF INFANTS. An infant is exercised by being carried and dandled in its nurse's arms, (but note this, that no dandling or violent motion must be allowed until the infant has strength to bear it,) by having its body and limbs well rubbed at the time of dressing and undressing. When sufficiently strong it ought to be placed upon the ground to roll about, and stretch its limbs ; when it begins actively to observe, its toys may be placed about it, and it will move about to collect them ;

let these toys, however, be of such a nature that if the child's
face should fall upon them, no material injury could take
place ; those of a circular form, such as a ball, a ring, a tam-
bour, and the like, are the best. I have known a child lose its
life by falling upon a small *drum-stick*, which, through the eye
penetrated the brain ; avoid, therefore, all angular toys, such
as whips, sticks, windmills, or even dolls, IF the legs be of
wood. When the child can walk a little, be careful to have it
well watched, and give strict injunctions that all accidents,
falls, &c., be reported to you, that you may examine it ; spinal
and other affections, which produce imbecility or deformity
have often arisen from the neglect of this attention.

9.—Every healthful infant should be vaccinated by the
seventh week, (to prevent the ravages of that fatal enemy to
beauty, the small-pox,) as this is the best time for the child to
receive it.

10.—We have advised that the child should sleep with its
mother ; we must now caution the mother against allowing the
infant to sleep at the breast ; it not only injures the beauty of
the breast, but injures the child ; for the first month, indeed,
the infant, if awake, may be put to the breast once in about
two or three hours ; but after that time, once in four hours is
sufficient ; but let it be done upon system, and not at irregular
intervals. The frequent taking of the breast in the night is
not only unnecessary and injurious, but if the child is habitua-
ted thereto, its rest will be broken and its digestion injured,
even if we say nothing of the mischief which broken rest is
calculated to produce upon the mother, who should also recollect that what injures her, injures her child, who derives its
support from her. Many a child has been suffocated by going
to sleep with the nipple in its mouth.

11.—We must not close our hints without impressing upon
mothers, the importance of giving the strictest orders, that the
eyes of the new-born infant be shielded from all light, natural
or artificial ; and, further, to be very particular in the choice
of their nurses ; let them not engage a noisy one, a gossiping,
a bustling, or a fidgety one, and let them avoid, as they would
a *cobra*, one of those kind old women who are so considerate
as to imagine, that the dear newly-made mamma is continually
in want of stimulants, to support her strength or to raise her
spirits.

12.—In conclusion, we would advise mothers not to press
their children to mental exertion until the sixth or seventh
year ; much information may, however, be imparted by visible
objects, without immediate application to the memory—(getting by heart, as it is called). If a child has an inclination to

learr, you need not thwart it; but experience proves, when mental exertion is rigidly enforced at an early age, that it frequently produces disease of the brain, water in the head, which, by destroying health, prevents the development of the various organs, mental and physical ; if but a temporary injury to the health from this unnatural exertion was sure to be accompanied by some equivalent improvement in the intellectual system, some persons might endeavor to justify the practice, but unfortunately, the reverse is usually the case, a very juvenile prodigy in intellectual acquisitions, seldom makes a great man and for this simple reason : the mind has been so overwrought by exertion before it attained strength to bear it, that in many cases the little sufferer has sunk into the grave ; and in others, after having attained a certain eminence above those of his age, from pure exhaustion he has stopped, and awaited their passing him without energy to prevent it; there are few persons who have lived much in the world, but must have observed that most of the *mediocres* of their acquaintance had, at one time, been considered prodigies.

CHAPTER II.

BEAUTY OF FORM.

REMARKS ON THE ANATOMICAL CONSTRUCTION OF THE HUMAN BODY—
DEFORMITIES PRODUCED BY CLOTHES, IN YOUTH—STAYS—ADVICE TO
MARRIED LADIES AS TO THE PRESERVATION OF THEIR SHAPE—POSI-
TION—STOOPING—PROPER DIRECTIONS FOR SECURING BEAUTY OF FORM.

WE shall now give a few remarks upon the anatomical construction of the human body. We present them because they
give such a view of the anatomical arrangement of the human
form, as will prove to the young mother the perfection of nature's work, and, we trust, induce her to resort to none of
those fashionable restrictions upon the operations of nature,
which, professing to assist, only destroy her power, or direct
it into an improper course. In the progress of the work we
shall point out, how nature may be assisted when she requires
assistance, and also how dangerous it is unnecessarily to tam-
per with her operations.

The general beauty of the human body, in all its features
and combinations, is calculated to excite the admiration and
wonder of mankind. Herein are contained the principles of
mechanical and optical science.

The skull, which is soft at birth, becomes elastic in childhood, and little liable to injury from concussion. The parts
which are most likely to be brought into violent contact, are
thick, while the sutures remain loose; but as maturity advances
and accidents become less frequent, *then* the bones lose that
nature, which would render concussion harmless—and the
timidity of *age* teaches man that his structure is no longer
adapted to active life. If a workman were to inspect the join-
ing of the bones of the cranium, he would admire the minute
dove-tailing by which one bone is inserted into and surrounded

by another, whilst that other pushes out its processes or jut-
tings between those of the first in the same manner, and thus
the fibres of the two become interlaced and strengthened. The
pressure to which the upper part of the skull is frequently subject, is provided for by the contrivance of cross bones, which
traverse the base of the skull, preventing the bones from being
driven out of their places on the one hand, or being drawn in-
ward on the other. The beauty of the framework, as exhibited in the spinal construction, is wonderfully interesting.
This organ consists of twenty-four bones, each bending a
little, and making a joint with its fellow—all yielding in a
slight degree, and permitting, in its whole line, that degree of
flexibility which is necessary to the motions of the body. Between these bones, or vertebræ, there is an elastic gristly substance, which permits them to approach, and play a little in
the actions of the body. Whenever a weight is upon the
head, this gristle yields; and the moment it is removed, the
gristle regains its place, and the bones resume their position.
The spine, which is in the form of an italic _f_, yields, recoils,
and forms the most perfect spring, calculated to carry the head
without jar or injury. The spine rests on what is called the
pelvis, a circle of bones, of which the haunches are the extreme parts.

Sir Charles Bell, in his popular Treatise on Animal Me-
chanics, (from which this information was originally taken,)
in speaking of the beautiful arrangement of the human frame,
observes, that he could undertake to prove that the foundation
of the Eddystone Lighthouse—the perfection of human archi-
tecture and ingenuity—is not formed on principles so correct
as those which have directed the arrangement of the bones of
the human foot; that the most perfect pillar, or king-post, is
not adjusted with the accuracy of the hollow bones, which support our weight; that the insertion of a ship's mast into the
hull is a clumsy contrivance, compared with the connexions of
the human spine and pelvis; and that the tendons are composed in a manner superior to the patent cables of Huddart, or
the yet more recently improved chain cables of Bloxam.

It has been said that the centre, or middle part, between the
extremities of the head and feet of a well-proportioned infant,
is the navel, but of an adult it is the os pubis; this, though not
absolutely correct, is so nearly so, as to deserve attention.
Artists, who make a daily study of the most perfect developments of the human figure, generally divide the measures of
children into four, five, or six parts, of which one is given to
the head. A child of two years old, is, in general, about five
heads high; of five years old, nearly six; about fifteen or six-

teen years of age, seven heads are the proportion of measure, and the centre declines to the upper part of the pubis. Hence it appears, that as the growth of the body advances, there is a gradual approach to the proportion of an adult of nearly eight heads—in the whole height of which, as before mentioned, the head itself makes one.

It is not, however, to be supposed that beauty is limited to any single shape or figure, and that a deviation from ordinary received notions of correct proportion must necessarily imply deformity. The forms of beauty in the human figure are as varied as the varieties of human genius. We should not wish to reduce the stature and form of a majestic beauty to the delicate figure of the Medicean Venus; nor to enlarge the proportions of the diminutive beauty to the classical dimensions of the Trojan Helen. These varieties have each their own peculiar charms ; each may be exquisite and perfect in itself, and unsurpassable within its own immediate sphere.

It has been doubted whether the human figure was ever seen in such perfect proportions as are developed in some of the statues of antiquity. Undoubtedly, the sculptor, when forming his *beau ideal* of beauty, never forms it from a single model :—one may supply a bust of perfect contour—a second a hand or arm—the leg and foot of a third are brought into his service ; and thus it is, by selecting their several beauties from many forms, that he is enabled to blend into one the representation of a perfect whole.

The foregoing extract will give some idea of the perfection of the machinery which supports the human body ; and we should think would convince the most skeptical how little nature can require from art in ordinary cases : if the reader will therefore bear in mind the true object of clothing, and abandon all restraints that do not affect this object, she will avoid many deformities to which nine women out of ten are subject, in the present artificial state of society. We will detail the objects of clothing.

1st. To protect the body from differences of temperature, and keep up a uniformity of the vital heat.

2d.—To assist nature in the development of stature, by supporting the body in its position, (when it requires support,) without by pressure interfering with the growth of the muscles and the circulation of the blood ; for the moment sufficient pressure is used to do this, you impede the efforts of nature instead of assisting her ; because, if by means of bands or stays, or any other mechanical contrivance, you cause pressure upon the muscles which support the body, you invariably diminish their size, and, of course, their strength. Not only do we most decidedly condemn tight stays, but also tight waistbands, sleeves, or, in short, any part of the apparel that acts upon the regular flow of the blood and development of muscle ; for if the blood is impeded in its course, reason must assure us that the muscles that are nourished by it must pine for want of nourishment, and that ultimately the body, from the weakness of these muscles, must gradually lose its proper position : nor is this the only injury which the figure sustains ; for, if pressure is applied in one part, it must force an unnatural growth in another, thereby producing a form never conceived by the great Author of nature. Look at the figure of a modern belle, with a waist like a spider, the bosom pressed into the neck, and the hips and haunches forced into unnatural elevation : then regard the exquisite form of the Venus de Medici, with its graceful curves—with no sudden depressions—but with one beauty gliding into another, perfection succeeding perfection, while the eye follows each untired, because ever changing, with no abrupt termination.

Did it never occur to my reader how completely the formation of the bows of the ribs are thus altered, and, by the alteration, how much the varied functions of nature must be impeded ; that debility, indigestion, consumption, and a general interruption of health, must be the consequences ; that the maternal functions are also most fearfully interfered with, and that she who perseveres in these monstrosities, adds tenfold to the ordinary danger of becoming a mother—that she adds bitterness indeed to the primitive curse : " I will greatly multiply thy sorrow and thy conception ; in sorrow thou shalt bring forth children ;" but we shall speak more on this head when we address ourselves to the injuries thus caused, to which, from its importance, we shall devote a separate chapter. We here wish to impress upon the minds of all who have the management of children and growing females, the great danger of tight dressing, and particularly of tight lacing ; we wish to show that this tightness does not even momentarily improve the figure, and that it is only by the ignorant, by persons without taste, that the wasp-like figure into which the shape of young girls is sometimes compressed, can be esteemed handsome or graceful. As we before said, let young ladies take the Venus de Medici as the example of what a figure should be—as that figure which every man of taste considers perfect ; and be assured that he will look upon her figure as approaching perfection in the proportion she approaches that ; a very small waist, unless the whole figure harmonizes therewith, is a deformity. This is not an opinion, it is a fact,—one that does not admit of dispute, which is referable to a standard from which there is no appeal. The great philosopher of the seventeenth century, who was also a medical man, remarks: "Whalebone stays often narrow the chest, render the back crooked, produce a tendency to consumption, promote indiges-, tion, and often render the breath fœtid." Is it then possible that my reader will persevere in the system of tight lacing, when the experience of the learned of all ages since its introduction has universally condemned the practice. It must, however, be recollected that, as mere artificial aids, we do not absolutely prohibit stays : we put our veto against steel busks in the most unqualified language ; we object to the introduction of whalebone, except very sparingly ; and wholly condemn that degree of lacing which can, by its pressure, affect the circulation of the blood, or flatten and prevent the growth of the muscles. What a shocking absurdity is it to see a young girl laced so tight, that she can scarcely breathe! what a disgraceful one to see her fainting under this self-inflicted injurious, and absurd torture! "What," says Mrs. Walker, "is the effect of this compression upon the eye and mind of the observer? It excites an instantaneous conviction of artifice, and a very natural suspicion of its necessity; notions equally at variance with beauty and purity are called up, and the object of these dark thoughts may excite much more contempt than admiration. When, indeed, a lady is tightly laced, she loses the character at once of beauty, of grace, and of innocence !!"

While we are on the subject of stays, &c., &c., we will give a few words of advice to married women on the preservation of their shape. And first be it observed that married women have a much greater probability of preserving their shape than old maids, provided they they take proper care of themselves ; and religiously abjure all extravagant pressure by stays, &c., &c. The organization of the female is such that the end of her existence is not answered unless she have children. An old maid, then, can scarcely be said to be in a state of nature. She necessarily is subject to a variety of suppressions, diseases, &c., &c., incidental to the uterine system when its proper functions are not called into operation ; and so marked is this effect, that nine times out of ten an old maid might be discovered by her countenance ; a beautiful old maid would be a *lusus naturæ*, for illness, consequent upon her position, excites the temper, and writes discontent upon the countenance, a fatal enemy this to beauty. Do not, however, let my reader suppose that we hold these antiquities in contempt ; many a valuable member of society has doomed herself to this description of isolation, not from want of natural affections,

but from their disappointment; not from coldness of heart but
from a broken spirit; thus exhibiting instances of pure devo-
tedness and self-sacrifice rarely to be found but in woman :
honor, then, be to old maids. To return, however, to our subject. Note then—

It has been the custom in many cases for pregnant women
to endeavor to conceal their size by having their stays made
particularly long, and tightly laced : from hence arises a fact
which cannot be too deeply impressed upon the mind, that
women who do so are generally larger in appearance than
those who do not, the enlargement arising from disease pro-
moted by the practice ; they are also much subject to hyste-
rics, sickness, and general debility, from the same cause ; the
child also will generally be either deformed, stunted in its
growth, or weakly in its constitution. These are the effects
of improper bandages. The mother does, however, require
certain supports, which her more experienced friends or her
medical attendant will recommend. To preserve the figure,
let it have proper support ; let the clothing fit the figure,
but not too tightly. After confinement, a little attention will
also be required. It was formerly the custom to bind the
mother with tight belts and bandages ; all that is now necessary will be done by the accoucheur. The muscles which
have been for months upon the stretch, will of course be re
laxed when relieved from the pressure of the infant; the
mother will therefore require some little support; but so long
as the horizontal position is maintained in bed, it is question-
able if much good is derived from it. When she begins to sit
up, it will, however, be highly necessary to retain the binder,
which has already, we will suppose, been supplied ; or a petti-
coat with a broad band, tied closely, but not too tight, will
answer the same end, by supporting the parts until their ordi
nary strength is restored.

Another popular error we will expose. Many ladies have
a notion that suckling tends to injure the beauty of the breast :
true, it may be made to do so, but only by the want of information, or the absence of energy in the mother. If, for instance,
when suckling, she allows the infant to hang, dragging as it
were, at the bosom, it will of course destroy the symmetry of
its form ; but if, during this operation, she holds the infant well
up to her, sitting upright rather than stooping, she will find no
such consequences,—the contrary, indeed, is the fact. Nature
prepares this food for the infant; if, therefore, it is not given,
the breast is necessarily distended and injured, and the process
of dispersing the milk at this unnatural period is often attended
with destructive consequences to beauty. Care should be

taken also to feed the child from both breasts, or one may become larger than the other. Some mothers also permit the child to lie at the breast all night—this is injurious, not only to the form of the mother, but to the child ; this bad habit is calculated to injure the digestion of the child, and to disturb the rest of both infant and mother. (See also Chap. I.)

Let the mother, then, attend to these directions, and we will insure her from any injury to her figure ; for she may depend that the duties of a mother are calculated to improve the form, until age, the great destroyer of beauty, demand the usual tribute to nature's imperative law.

Position. Much injury is, without doubt, done to the figures of young ladies from the ordinary routine of their education : in learning the harp, to write, to draw, the attention of the mother, or the governess, ought to be particularly directed to the position of the pupil; in each of these employments the left shoulder is very apt to be depressed. Let a book, of sufficient thickness to equalize the height of the shoulders, be placed under the left arm, and it will be found that this very simple contrivance will much tend to remedy the tendency in the two latter employments : fortunately for our fair readers, the harp is not commonly much practised until the form is in some degree set ; nevertheless, we particularly direct the attention to the possible consequences of its practice.

Domestic habits will frequently tend, also, to draw the figure upon one side. If, for instance, a young girl always sits, in her ordinary employments upon one side of the fireplace, or the window ; if she accustoms herself to lie upon one side only in bed,—she will most likely find that, imperceptibly, on one side the muscles have enlarged, strengthened, and drawn down that side—that upon the other they have become lax, and yielded to the strong power of the other. Let it be borne in mind, that all our powers are improved by use, that pressure, continually applied to one part, impairs the strength of the muscles, and, by diminishing their volume, weakens them. Many persons acquire a habit of stooping ; this may be occasioned by a variety of causes,—by certain employments, or by a feeling of weakness in the chest or in the back ; indulgence in this habit, however, in either case, increases the evil. We shall, therefore, without stopping to investigate the cause, recommend the following advice, which, some years since, was given by a popular writer :

" That I may be more clearly understood," says he, " it will be necessary to inform my unprofessional readers, that the part of the back formed by the ribs is not a flat, but a round surface,

and, as the shoulder-blades rest on this, they would fall either
forwards or towards the spine, were there not some means of
keeping them in a proper position. They are most disposed
to fall forwards ; for, although the collar-bones appear to hold
them back, these bones are united to the breast-bone by a
movable joint, and, as the weight of the arms operates prin-
cipally on the anterior angles of the shoulder-blades, both the
collar-bones and the shoulders would fall forwards, were it not
for the action of several strong muscles, which pass from the
spine to the shoulder-blade. But these muscles may be destroyed by any contrivance that supersedes their use, which
the back-board most certainly does ; for, if the shoulder-blades
be brought close to the spine by the straps of the collar, and
kept constantly so, there can be no use for the muscles, which
ought to bind them ; they must, from want of exercise, waste
and become useless, or nearly so, while those on the fore part
of the chest, being excited to resistance, will increase in power,
and whenever the collar is removed will drag the shoulders
forward ; while the relaxed muscles behind will give way in an
equal degree, having been so reduced in tension, by want of
exercise, that they become inert and yielding. We should
therefore recommend that, instead of a person who stoops putting on a back-board and bracing back the shoulders, thereby
increasing the evil, that he should endeavor to increase the
power of the muscles behind by resistance ; and we cannot il-
lustrate our meaning better, perhaps, than by suggesting the
practice of carrying a weight in front, suspended by a strap
from the back of the neck, in the manner of the Turkish Jews
who frequent the streets of London, and whose erect figures
are, in some measure, so many proofs of the correctness of our
views of the subject."   An eminent surgeon related to me the
following anecdote, which, as it may be useful to the reader, I
have here quoted :—

   " He was consulted by a gentleman, who is now one of our
first tragedians, as to the best mode of correcting a stoop which
he had acquired.   Our friend told him that neither stays nor
straps would do him any essential good, and that the only
method of succeeding, was to recollect to keep his shoulders
braced back by a voluntary effort.   But the tragedian replied,
that this he could not do, as his mind was otherwise occupied.
The surgeon then told him that he could give him no further
assistance.   Shortly after this conversation, this actor ordered
his tailor to make a coat of the finest kerseymere, so as to fit
him very tightly when his shoulders were thrown back.
Whenever his shoulders fell forward, he was reminded by a
pinch under the arms that his coat cost him six guineas, and

that it was made of very fragile materials. Being thus forced, for the sake of his fine coat, to keep his shoulders back, he soon cured himself of the stoop. My friend was much obliged to him for the hint, and afterwards, when consulted whether young ladies should wear shoulder straps, permitted them on condition that they were made of fine muslin, or valuable silk, for tearing which there should be a forfeit."

In conclusion, we most decidedly condemn all descriptions of machines or braces which are so applied as to restrain the shoulders, or to press heavily on any one part of the female form ; the former in particular must keep up an unnatural stretch of those muscles which move the arms and shoulders forward, and of course must reduce that plumpness of the upper part of the chest, which is so indispensable to elegance of shape, while it forces at the same time the breast-bone to protrude below, and press inwards above, impeding the free play of the lungs, tainting the breath, and leading directly to consumption. In the second place, it must keep in a most unnatural contraction the muscles which move the arms and shoulders backwards, and as this contraction is never relieved so long as the braces are worn, the muscles rapidly diminish in size and strength, and when the braces are laid aside, the shoulders must fall forward for want of support, and the deformity is probably rendered from the continuance of the practice, almost, if not altogether incurable. From the want of motion also and proper exercise in these muscles, the flow of the blood to that part of the chest will be greatly diminished, and the ribs and bones of the chest, which, like other parts of the body, depend on the blood for their nourishment, must suffer for the want of their natural supply, and will become smaller, and from feebleness will lose the fine arched form that constitutes the beauty of the female bust. In a word, the chicken breast will ensue, with all its threatening consequences of cough and fatal consumption.

We caution mothers most strongly not to be deceived by the apparent improvement they produce when first put on ; for this is the snare that has allured so many to torture their children into deformity. Follow the example of the elegant Greeks, the ease and beauty of whose forms are so much admired. They put no unnatural straps on their young ladies , all their garments were easy, loose, and floating ; and the effects were seen in their every limb, and their every motion. On the contrary, we can at once distinguish among thousands, from their stiff, starched awkwardness, the poor creatures who have been pinioned and tortured by shoulder-straps and other wicked inventions to turn beauty into deformity, and the finest figures into rickety ugliness.   Dr. Macartney, of **Dublin,** says he has found the fine proportions of the antique statues only in the busts of women who had never worn such restraints on shape.   How very extraordinary, then, must be the infatuation, which, in spite of the experience of all practical men— in spite of the torment to which these instruments subject their wearers until habit has rendered them bearable : how strong must be the impulse, that will induce ladies to continue to wear them.

    Of the consequences of pressure from stays, &c., we **shall give** the details in the next chapter.

CHAPTER III.

BEAUTY OF FORM

DESTROYED BY TIGHT LACING—MRS. WALKER'S ILLUSTRATION OF THE FACT.

THE evils of tight lacing are all but incredible. Mr. Coulson, in his work upon the "Deformities of the Chest and Spine," enumerates ninety-seven diseases which frequently do, and always may arise from this cause ; among them are, apoplexy—hunchback—cancer in the breast—asthma—consumption—disease of the heart—liver complaint—premature labor—difficult and protracted labor—miscarriage—hernia—and epileptic fits. This list, one would think, should suffice to frighten any lady from this diabolical habit. He however adds, that it usually causes "a sickly and short life," and not unfrequently "unhealthy children, ugly children, and the birth of monstrosities."

To press the subject still more upon the attention of my fair readers, I make the following quotation from Mrs. Walker's work, entitled, "Female Beauty :"—

"The human form has been moulded by nature, and the best shape is undoubtedly that which she has given it. To endeavor to render it more elegant by such means, is to change it : to make it much smaller below, and much larger above, is to destroy its beauty ; to keep it cased up in a kind of domestic cuirass, is not only to deform it, but to expose the internal parts to numerous and frightful accidents. Under this compression, the development of the bones, which arc still tender, does not take place conformably to the intentions of nature ; because nutrition is stopped, and they consequently become twisted and deformed. Soemmerring, in one of his works, presents us a drawing made from nature, of the figure of a woman who had all her life worn tight stays, and one of the statue of the Medicean Venus ; and nothing can better exemplify the horrible effects of this absurd practice."

Women who wear very tight stays complain that they cannot sit upright without them ; nay, are sometimes compelled to wear night stays when in bed, and this strikingly proves to what an extent tight stays weaken the muscles of the trunk. It is this which disposes to lateral curvature of the spine. From these facts, as well as many others, it is evident, that tight stays, far from preventing the deformities, more or less considerable, which an experienced eye might remark among ninety out of every hundred young girls, are, on the contrary, the cause of these deviations. Stays, therefore, should never be worn under any circumstances, till the organs have acquired a certain development ; and they should never at any period be tigl... A well known effect of the use of stays is, that the right shoulder frequently becomes larger than the left, because the former being stronger and more frequently in motion, somewhat frees itself, and acquires by this means an increase, of which the left side is deprived, by being feebler and subjected to continued compression. " The injury," says a correspondent of the Scotsman, " does not fall merely on the internal structure of the body, but also on its beauty, and on the temper and feelings with which that beauty is associated. Beauty is in reality but another name for that expression of countenance, which is the index of sound health, intelligence, good feelings, and peace of mind. All are aware that uneasy feelings, existing habitually in the breast, speedily exhibit their signature on the countenance, and that bitter thoughts, or a bad temper, spoil the human face divine of its grace. But it is not so generally known that irksome or painful sensations, though merely of a physical nature, by a law equally certain, rob the temper of its sweetness, and as a consequence, the countenance of the more ethereal and better part of its beauty. In many persons, tight stays displace the breast, and produce an ineffaceable and frightful wrinkle between it and the shoulder. And in others whom nature has not gifted with the plumpness necessary to beauty, such stays make the breasts still flatter and smaller. Generally speaking, tight stays destroy also the firmness of the breast, sometimes prevent the full development of the nipples, and give rise to those indurations of the mammary glands, the cause of which is frequently not well understood, and which are followed by such dreadful consequences.

" They also cause a reddish tinge of the skin, swelling of the neck, &c. A delicate and slender figure is full of beauty

.n a young person; but suppleness and ease confer an additional charm. Yet most women, eager to be in the extreme of fashion, lace themselves in their stays as tight as possible, and undergoing innumerable tortures, appear stiff, ungraceful, and ill-tempered. Elegance of shape, dignity of movement, grace of manner, and softness of demeanor, are all sacrificed to foolish caprice. Stays tend to transform into a point the base of the cone, which the osseous frame of the chest represents, and to maintain in a state of immobility two cavities, whose dimensions should vary without ceasing. By this compression stays are prejudicial to the free execution of several important functions, muscular motion, circulation, respiration, digestion. The muscles or organs of motion are enlarged by free exercise, and are destroyed by compression; every degree of this as exercised by stiff stays, diminishes and enfeebles the muscles of the chest; a great degree of it absolutely annihilates them. Long before that is accomplished, the stays become necessary for support instead of the muscles; but as their support is remote from the spine, as well as inadequate, it yields, and lateral curvature, or crooked back ensues. Retreat to natural habits is now difficult or impossible; if the muscles retain any power, they increase the curvature, and the wretched being is reduced to the necessity of obtaining support, and maintaining existence, by stays still stiffer during the day, and at night, by stays when in bed. By impeding the circulation of blood through the lungs, the use of stays not only prevents their proper development, and renders respiration difficult, but becomes a predisposing cause of convulsive coughs, consumption, palpitation of the heart, and aneurism. From the same cause, obstinate and dangerous obstructions in the abdominal organs, which are displaced by the pressure of the .busk, are of frequent occurrence. In females, the liver has frequently been found pushed several inches beyond the last ribs, and its superior surface perceptibly marked with them; and this produced solely by the pressure of the stays upon the organs contained in the chest. The breasts, owing to compression, are, as well as other organs, liable to become scirrhous; and an opening is thus made for cancerous affections and hysterical diseases, to which last a sedentary life alone sufficiently predisposes Difficult labors, and the utter wreck which they produce of health and of beauty, are equally the effects of the hip or haunch bones being altered during youth by the pressure of stays."

In addition to the above authority, I may add, that White and Doering have detailed cases in which tight corsets have actually displaced the womb: and M Desormeaux, of Paris

cites many cases in which tight lacing has produced dangerous
and sometimes fatal cases of inflammation both of the breasts
and womb : indeed, what will injure the one is generally followed by injury to the other ; a fact which should induce
mothers never to wear anything tight over the breast during
pregnancy ; for this will tend to retard the growth of the fœtus,
by deranging the functions of the uterus (womb), and may be
the cause of innumerable deformities in the child.

When we reflect upon the many evils to which stays and
corsets give rise, and notice of what little utility they are—
when we examine the construction of the female form, and observe the exquisite beauty of its contour, as nature perfected
it, we almost wish for the resurrection of Joseph II., who for-
bad their use in all public charities and in all convents over
which he had command ; and further, to make the wearing of
them disgraceful, he ordered " that all women who were condemned by the laws to corporeal punishment, should wear stays
and hoops." Will our readers believe it, that even this did not
entirely abolish the custom ! ! !

CHAPTER IV.

BEAUTY OF FORM.

HABITS FAVORABLE TO THE DEVELOPMENT OF BEAUTY—TRAINING—EARLY
RISING —EXERCISE—CLOTHING — MEALS — CORPULENCE — LEANNESS OF
BREASTS AND BODY.

FROM its very great importance we have already devoted
considerable space to the subject of this chapter, and have endeavored to prove that the figure cannot but be injured by confinement of any sort, from the simple fact, which is not capable
of contradiction—viz., that the pressure upon any part of the
form must prevent its growth, must therefore injure the healthi-
ness of the subject; and by unnaturally contracting one part,
force an unnatural growth upon another : it is a well-known
truth among surgeons, that the fine proportions of the antique
statues are only to be found in the busts of women who have
never submitted to these unnatural restraints.   We are most
anxious to impress this upon the minds of our fair readers
being certain, that if they will give a trial to our directions
their figures, if not already perfect, must be improved ; but
unless they at once abandon their lacing our task is hopeless ;
for there is no habit not absolutely immoral, which more immediately injures the complexion, as well as the figure, as does
tight compression.

We have spoken of the injury the general form and health
receive from certain habits ; we must now notice that even in
spinal affections, bandages must only be resorted to under the
advice of an experienced medical man.   The mother's best
plan, in such cases, is to go at once to a first-rate practitioner ;
it would be cruel in us to make her believe, that however
perfect our theory, she could cure a radical defect in the form
of her child, without medical superintendence.

"HEALTH ' as we have several times said, "is the fountain

of Beauty ;" we shall now give such directions as will promote the general health, and detail such a procedure as will, under ordinary circumstances, secure the beauty of the form, and much improve any complexion. Special directions respecting the complexion are, however, given in the next chapter.

HABITS FAVORABLE TO THE DEVELOPMENT OF BEAUTY.— Going to bed and rising early, are lessons which nature teaches, and which we must insist upon, if our readers wish to preserve their charms in perfection ; they can never be out of bed later than 10 o'clock, P. M., nor in bed after 6, A. M., in the summer, without retarding the operation of our directions if they are in moderate health : most females require eigh hours' sleep, nor do we recommend them to take less ; but it must never be forgotten, that too much sleep, instead of refreshing, produces a desire for still further indulgence ; it has the effect of long privation of exercise upon the mental and muscular organs ; it destroys the complexion, and is even vitally injurious—for it relaxes the whole organization of the body, produces a disposition to paralysis, and thus often is the unsuspected cause of death. These facts will give our readers some idea of the effects of too much sleep ; but while we condemn the habit of taking too much sleep, we must not forget that want of sleep will bring on premature old age : lying awake, at night, is highly injurious ; it causes a rapid evaporation of organic particles, and prevents their being replaced in the system ; consequently, it has the effect of hastening the progress of life, in other words, of shortening life ; this will be the result, whether the loss of sleep be voluntary or involun tary ; let not therefore our fair readers be led away by the popular idea, which indeed has been propagated by many who ought to know better--viz. : that every hour stolen from sleep is so much added to the length of existence ; improper abstraction from the hours of sleep will, on the contrary, shorten life. We will now refer to the proper time for sleep.

It is a common observation, that one hour's sleep before twelve o'clock is worth two after twelve. There is much truth in the saying : people must not therefore imagine that it matters not whether they have the proper quantity of sleep by night or by day, so that they have it : the reason that sleep before twelve at night is so beneficial, is obvious. Any physician will inform our readers, that all persons have, or ought to have, once in the twenty-four hours, a critical perspiration ; this is very conspicuous in some subjects, and though scarcely perceptible in others, it is not the less efficacious. By this, whatever useless or injurious particles are in our bodies, are emoved ; this diurnal crisis is absolutely necessary to health and the proper period for it is when the sun is in the nadir, or twelve o'clock at night. If awake, we are all sensible of the presence of the fever which brings on this crisis, by feeling a less disposition to sleep, a temporary activity both of mind and body, and this is particularly observable in very nervous persons. Those persons, therefore, who make this a means to enable them to bear increased exertion, whether in the pursuit of pleasure, or business, are completely frustrating the designs of nature; they will never have a perfect crisis—the secretions of the body will never be properly removed—decay of health, destruction of complexion, a premature old age, will certainly be the consequence. Such misconduct is, then, a most fatal enemy to beauty. The injury to health and to complexion arising from late hours, is not however confined to the destructive consequences arising from an habitually imperfect crisis; those who rise late lose all the advantages of the solar light and heat; and of the more inspiring, because more oxygenated air of the morning. Morning is the time for the exercise of the intellect; the mind is then clear, and the body receives an extraordinary exhilaration from inhaling the new air of the young hours of day. Never do we enjoy so completely a sense of intellectual existence, as when we welcome by our presence the infant streaks of morning.

But some of our readers may say, Sleep is not always to be obtained; we would be early risers, but we cannot sleep of a night, or until the approach of morning; consequently, we are unable to rise early. We are willing to allow that there are but few who have not, at some time or another, been desirous of attaining sleep, and still unable to do so; we will therefore give a means of obtaining sleep whenever it is desired, provided always, that neither the body nor the mind are under the influence of that degree of pain, which will render it impossible to attend to our directions.

RECIPE.—Place yourself in bed in that position which you know to be most favorable to sleep. Let there be no light in the room, nor any noise to distract the attention; then take a deep respiration. The breath thus drawn into the lungs must not be discharged through the mouth, (which must be closed,) but gently through the nostrils. If the mouth be kept closed, this hard respiration will then be succeeded involuntarily by a number of smaller ones; all these must be discharged, if I may so say, through the nostrils; but from first to last you must direct the closed eyes and the mental vision toward the nose, watching, as it were, the breath coming therefrom at each respiration; endeavor to keep the mind intently on this act for a quarter of an hour, and we will guarantee you shall not be aware of the extent to which your task has been performed, for you will be asleep before the time has expired ; *mental vision must, however, be employed in the act, and you must not be discussing the probability of its success : for it is to the isolation of thought that this employment secures, that you will be indebted for its success.* The philosophy of the act is very simple, viz. : in *perfect* sleep the mind is absolutely at rest (*not dreaming*) ; if it be confined to one thought, it is in that state which is the nearest approach to sleep ; and when wearied by the act of isolation, the bounds between active life and the image of death are quickly passed, as our readers will soon find, if they determinedly follow our directions.

We will now say a few words on the position which is most adapted to prevent injury to the form when lying in bed, and thus prevent the "sweet restorer of nature" from being a means of injuring the form. Common sense will tell us that an unnatural position long sustained must produce an injurious effect upon the spine : any person will also be liable to organic injury by lying always on the same side. The position therefore should be changed every night, or at any time, if awake, during the night. Instances have been known of the internal parts of the chest and abdomen growing together from being brought into continual contact. The horizontal position of the body should be nearly preserved ; the pillow in ordinary cases should not be high, but when a high pillow is necessary, the line from the head to the foot should be scarcely broken. This my reader will see is all but impossible, if feather or down beds are laid upon ; in these the loins are apt to sink into the bed, the shoulder is pushed out of its place, the chin is forced into the chest, the neck is twisted, as shown in the sketch (in plate No. 3) ; all these are, of course, highly injurious to the shape. Down and feather beds also retain the exhalations from the body with so much pertinacity, that except by exposure to a fire or hot air, they can seldom be thoroughly eradicated ; such beds, consequently, are fearful sources of cold, rheumatism, and consumption.

Instead therefore of a feather or down bed, we recommend a hair mattress ; with this, the indulgence of a down or feather pillow may be allowed ; when however it is necessary to keep the head high, as before said, care should be taken that a regular and gradual inclination of the form from the head downwards should be preserved, and that the loins do not sink : if the head be so raised as to place the body in a half-sitting posture, the effect will be highly injurious ; the circulation in the abdomen will be checked, and the spine compressed, the effect of which we have already shown.

The place of sleep must next be spoken of : it ought to be quiet, and without anything to attract the attention ; hence the impropriety of burning a light : this is correct in the abstract, but many nervous persons, who have contracted the habit of having a light burning during the night, would be so much excited by abandoning the habit, as to sustain more injury than the absence of the light would do good. To such we say, continue the light, but place it so in the shade as not to attract your attention. The bed-room ought to be large and airy : the windows ought to be kept open until sunset ; and it ought not to be either inhabited or heated during the day. In summer time, the door of the bed-room should be placed open as soon as the windows are shut on the approach of evening.

We have now to consider what are the best methods to secure beauty of form. What we are about to say must be taken in connection with what has already been said. The best methods are then the following :—Rise, and go to bed early—use a proper diet—avoid all improper bandages—take proper exercise—attend to the state of the digestive organs, and the form will improve, as the health must improve. We will, however, elaborate our ideas, and place them in a form, which we will call

TRAINING.—Before commencing our system, we would advise our readers to take the following mixture for three to seven days ; and as it has in its combination a slight aperient, the state of the uterine system must be regarded before taking it.

Carbonate of ammonia, 2 scruples,
Carbonate of soda, 2 drachms,
Infusion of senna comp., 2 ounces,
Infusion of gentian, 6 ounces.
Take two table spoonsful three times a day.

The character of the mixture is slightly stimulant, antacid, tonic, and mildly aperient ; and in forty-nine cases out of fifty must be beneficial. Whether it is so, may be judged after taking it for a day ; it usually raises the spirits, clears the mind, and strengthens the system ; the first two effects wil be very shortly felt.

After thus preparing the system, we recommend the following mode of procedure. Be it understood, however, that we are supposing the person to be in a state of ordinary good health, and affected by no chronic disorder. Under these circumstances, then, we can assure our readers that the training shall improve the complexion, give brightness to the eyes, and tone and strength to the system. We engage that it shall add ten years of freshness to the fading charms, and that it shall improve those which have youth for it to act upon.

Go to bed at ten o'clock, and if you have been long accustomed to late hours, commence by rising at seven, and each morning rise a quarter of an hour earlier, until you get up at half-past five. If you are able to walk from one to three miles before breakfast without fatigue, do so, and endeavor to employ the mind by the way, as this generally prevents fatigue. If at first you feel weary, walk in a garden with some friend for an hour, but do not stand about, keep up sufficient motion to prevent chilliness, and when you come in from your walk, if you have perspired, CHANGE YOUR CLOTHES, and let your person be well rubbed from ten to twenty minutes with a flesh brush, or hair gloves, (Dinneford's are the best,) particularly over the stomach and loins. When perfectly dry, put on a portion of your clothes, then wash your hands and face in cold water, and complete your dress ; all of which we presume has been changed if damped by perspiration. This is of vital importance ; also note, that no part of dress which has been damped by perspiration must be reworn till it has been well aired by THE FIRE ; mere exposure to the air will not do.

The breakfast must not be later than eight ; it may consist of a cup of strong tea, or coffee, if it agree with you, but not more ; a mutton chop, or a piece of steak, no fat, and if you can eat it underdone, the better ; with this you may eat a captain's biscuit, or dry toast WELL TOASTED ; the latter is best.

After breakfast, walk again ; on all occasions, however, endeavor to have an object in your walk, or some person with you to converse with ; as before said, this prevents fatigue, and consequently that lassitude of feeling and of countenance which, if long indulged, will leave its seal impressed upon the face, and thus be a bar to the production of beauty ; about three hours after breakfast you may take a biscuit, with a glass of sound ale, if it agree with you ; some constitutions will not bear malt liquor, but in general, exercise in the open air will soon so strengthen the system, as to enable it to do so ; if you do not take the ale, a glass of good old sherry wine may be taken, or a table spoonful of brandy in about a wine glass and a half of water. The forenoon, be it understood, must be spent in some active amusement.

Dine at half-past one ; your dinner must consist of a chop or steak ; now and then a roasted chicken may be allowed ; but one of the former must be the ordinary food ; a mealy potato may also occasionally be allowed ; but no pastry, puddings, made dishes, or *bon bons* of any sort ; a little thoroughly ripe fruit, (an hour or a little more after dinner,) may be taken occasionally, but had better be left alone ; a table spoon-ful of brandy in two wine glasses of water may be drunk with your dinner, if one glass of sound ale will not agree with you.

Take tea at from five to half-past, let it be one slice of dry toast, and ONE cup of good strong black tea ; there is no objection to the use of GOOD BUTTER in *moderation,* but it is better avoided until the system has experienced the benefit of this training.

Sup at eight. It may consist of a chop, cold roast mutton or beef ; in no case any fat ; a biscuit or dry toast may be eaten with it, and half a pint of ale ; or brandy and water as before directed. An hour's exercise ought to be taken after supper.

Let it never be forgotten, that at rising in the morning the whole of the person must be passed over with a sponge, dipped in lukewarm water ; (as soon as you can bear it, use cold water ;) that after being perfectly dried, the whole body from head to foot should then be well rubbed from ten to fifteen minutes with a flesh-brush, or one of Dinneford's hair gloves. If you have no person peculiarly attached to your service, one of the hair belts will be found most convenient, as all parts of the shoulders and back can then be reached. The same process must be pursued at night ; and the result will be such as no person can believe who has not tried it ; the skin will become soft, smooth, and in many cases almost transparent ; the muscles become firm, and the blood be diffused over the whole body ; this process prevents colds, chilblains, chapped hands, and assists digestion.

REMARKS UPON THE ABOVE SYSTEM OF TRAINING.—We have given a system of training, which will be applicable to ninety-nine cases out of every hundred. At the same time there are exceptions. Some, for instance, cannot walk without first taking refreshment ; such may be allowed half a cup of strong coffee, and a small slice of dry toast before starting on their walk. In other cases, malt liquor or sherry produces acidity of the stomach ; cold brandy and water may in such cases be substituted.*

* We must not, however, allow more brandy than the quantity specified ; to say nothing to the fact of its nullifying our system, it may lead to the filthy habit of taking brandy at all times, with or without necessity ; and a lady guilty of this sort of indiscretion can only excite *emotions of disgust* even if she had the graces of Venus, and the voice of Apollo. As we are on this subject, we must also warn our readers (speaking professionally) of the effect of this habit on the uterine system, which it cannot fail completely to disorganize,

We have directed the person training to take a strong diet, and much exercise. The state of the bowels and the uterine system must, however, be attended to. A lavement now and then, taken by means of Dr. Scott's apparatus, consisting of about a pint of warm water, will generally keep the bowels in regular order; (this must be attended to ;) or the following, if the water does not produce the desired effect.

Epsom salts, 2 ounces,
Castor oil, 2 ounces,
Warm water, 1 pint.

In some cases thin gruel is better than warm water. A very good lavement is composed of two table spoonsful of common salt (chloride of sodium) in a pint of warm water. (See Appendix, *Lavements.*)

These may be taken with advantage about half an hour after breakfast, when the bowels require attention. But warm water is usually quite sufficient for ordinary cases.

We have before referred to the state of the uterine system, but we say little upon the subject; for, without going more into details than could be allowed in a work of this kind, we could do little good ; our advice is, in any serious disorganization refer to your medical man ; but in ordinary cases, as the general health improves, that part of the system will improve also.

Our readers must not be alarmed, if for a week after they commence this system, they are a little feverish, or occasionally have a slight headache ; let them persevere, and they will feel the advantage of it.

We must caution them, however, against drinking between meals ; even if they are thirsty this must be avoided ; washing the hands and face frequently in cold water, will generally remove thirst, and this is the best way to do so, if thirsty between meal times.

Before closing this chapter, we must say a few words upon obesity, which, when it arrives at a certain state, is by medical men termed *polysarchia ;* and upon leanness, which is equally an enemy to beauty.

Corpulence is a disease that sometimes proves fatal. The difficulty of breathing with which very corpulent people are oppressed, is caused by an accumulation of fat on the kidneys, which obstructs the motion of the diaphragm ; whilst the heart

producing those weaknesses which are sources of so much annoyance to some females; it also destroys the complexion, produces fœtidity of the breath, and is the parent of very many of the ills which are consequent upon an artificial state of society.

ar.d large blood vessels being equally encumbered, a slowness
of pulse is produced, and possibly apoplexy and death. Corpulence generally arises from indulgence of the appetite, or in
taking too much sleep. In ordinary cases, our system of
training will remove it. But, in robust habits, we must alter
the diet, or increase the exercise ; we prefer the latter ; and,
in addition, let the person lie on a horse-hair mattress, and not
sleep more than six hours—say from 10 p.m. to 4 a.m. Strong
exercise, succeeded by change of clothes when perspiration
has been produced, with considerable friction of the skin at
each change of apparel, and morning and evening as before
directed, will usually prevent excessive corpulence. If, however, it fail, a vegetable diet must be adopted. All butter,
cream, beer, wine, and spirits must be abandoned, except that
quantity of brandy allowed for meals as before directed ; this
system, with exercise, (if possible in the open air,) and in the
intervals of exercise, having the mind properly applied, will,
we engage, reduce any ordinary case of obesity, and make the
individual active both in mind and body. When this is effected,
the return to animal food must be gradual, and the state of the
stomach and bowels must be attended to.

Many ladies who are not troubled with general obesity of
the system, have a superabundant development of the breast ;
the modern mode of reducing this is by a preparation of iodine ·
but as this is a dangerous internal medicine in unprofessiona.
hands, we shall recommend its external use, thus : Take

Iodine of zinc,—1 drachm,
Hog's lard,—1 ounce ;

mix well, and rub daily into each breast a piece about the size
of a nutmeg, a linen bandage so placed as gently to compress
the breast, without pressing upon the nipple, will assist its operation. We need scarcely say, this must not be done during
lactation or pregnancy.

Some of the old practitioners recommend pounded mint applied to the breasts, to check their exuberant growth, accompanied with bandages ; but to bandages, as a general rule, we
decidedly object ; when necessary, they must be used with
care, as just stated.

LEANNESS, when accompanied with decrease of strength,
must also arise from disease, and we recommend attention to
the general health, as it may be the herald of consumption ;
but if no decrease of strength accompanies it, though not a disease, it is still an enemy to beauty, as all angular development
is in opposition to gracefulness of figure. We must therefore
adopt a system totally opposed to that of our TRAINING, if we
wish to produce that approach to *embonpoint* which is

sary i) the beautiful. A diet at once nourishing and **strength**
ening, little exercise, from ten to twelve hours sleep, (say
from 10 p.m till 9 a.m.) A soft bed, complete tranquillity of
mind, little excitement, even of a pleasurable character, good
mild ale at dinner and supper, (but abstinence from spirits of
all sorts,) cream at breakfast and tea, with plenty of sugar, is
necessary to the accomplishment of our object. If the bosom
participates in the general leanness, its growth may be encou-
raged by having it loosely clothed, avoiding all pressure ; and
friction by the hand for an hour or two every day will assist
much in its development ; but *nothing* will more effectually
prevent it, than the artificial padding usually worn to supply
the natural deficiency, except indeed it be the artificial bosom,
said to be made of Indian-rubber, but which we only speak of
from report; this would most effectually stop their growth,
destroy its complexion, and probably produce disease, by a
complete exclusion of the air, and repression of the natural exhalations.

    We shall have much more to say upon the use of water and
friction in the chapters upon beauty of the skin and complexion

CHAPTER V.

BEAUTY OF THE COMPLEXION.

BEAUTY OF THE SKIN—COMPLEXION—CONSTRUCTION OF THE SKIN—IMPORT-
ANT FUNCTIONS OF — CARE OF — FRECKLES — WRINKLES—SUN-BURN—
BIRTH-MARKS—MOLES.

HAVING found in a work now but little known, a condensed description of the construction of the skin, we have incorporated it in the following remarks, retaining, however, our own views when we differ from the writer, and adding some important points of information, of which his account was deficient.

The skin is composed of three different coats, or layers, known as the outer, the middle, and the inner. The outer, or scarf skin, is nearly transparent,—as is seen when it is blistered,—and appears to be a most elaborate and delicately constructed net-work. It is extremely thin, except on such parts of the frame as are exposed to constant friction and labor—such as the palms of the hands and the soles of the feet: *even in infancy, this is the case.* The outer skin is insensible—as it does not contain nerves or veins—and is the only part of the body, except the teeth, which is fitted to endure direct exposure to the external air. During the continuance of vitality, moisture will pass through it, both outwards and inwards; but, after death, this faculty ceases. This outer skin is continually shed, whence the scurf which is found on the head, and may be plainly seen within black silk stockings, after they have been worn.

The membrane of color ;—under the scarf skin is a mucous net-work, which forms a soft bed to sheath the termination of the nerves in the inner skin, to prevent their being too keenly affected by external impressions ; and it is said that this layer is changed into scarf skin, when that has been destroyed. The inner surface of this mucous net-work is the seat of the small-pox and other eruptions, and abounds more in vessels and nerves than does the middle and outer surface; when these surfaces change into scarf skin they lose their vascularity. It is also the seat of color; and this fact has given rise to much speculation as to whether Negroes, Hindoos, and Europeans are of the same species—this membrane being absent in Albi- nos ; in Europeans not separable, as a continuous membrane ; and in Negroes it is distinctly continuous.

The true or innermost skin, is considerably thicker than the other two. On some parts of the body, this coating is much thinner than others ; more particularly on the eye-lids— through which, when closed, a bright light may be visible. On the lips, also, this layer is very thin, indeed nearly transpa- rent. The texture is extremely close and fibrous, abounding with minute pores, glands, and vessels, as well as the termina- tions of the nerves. These pores are so exquisitely minute, that a grain of sand is said to cover 25,000 ; they are used to receive moisture from without, as well as to carry off the insensible perspiration. In surgical operations, the cutting through this skin is always considered the most painful process. The skin being fibrous and spongy, is capable of contraction or distension ; any irritating substance applied to the surface will increase the size of the vessels, and create a superficial redness ; while the operation of cold, or of certain passions of the mind, will occasion the surface to dry, and present small raised portions, commonly called goose-skin.

When the skin is perfectly dry, the sense of touching is con- siderably impaired ; moisture is essential to vitality and sensa- tion, as well in this as in the enjoyment of the other senses. This moisture, prepared under the true skin, appears soft and soapy, and is separated from the blood by minute glands, whence it oozes to the surface. Independent of these glands there is an ointment given out to the skin, from the fat—parti- cularly where there is any hair. This frequently emits an un- pleasant smell,—which may be corrected by constant ablutions and perfumes.

The process of perspiration is always going on in the healthy subject, as may be discovered by holding any highly polished surface near the skin, such as a glass, which will very shortly become dimmed and steamed. This moisture will soil the linen, notwithstanding every precaution ; and, in some in- stances, it is said to be colored by the beverage, particularly by port wine, when taken freely. It is increased by exertion, and is then visible in drops ; and, being mingled with the oil of the skin, it is often of an unpleasant odor, particularly under the arm-pits, where this oil is the most abundant.

Between the vessels of the liver which separate the bile

from the blood, and the skin, there exists the strongest com-
panionship of any in the body. We cannot of course here go
into the particulars of the disorders of the liver and the bile,
but so much does the state of the skin depend or the healthi-
ness of the liver, that we hesitate not to say, that no washes,
nor external applications, can give permanent beauty to the skin,
until the digestive organs be freed from disorder, and all liver
and bilious complaints be removed. It is well known that
perspiration and the formation of bile proceed uniformly together, at all ages and in all climates. As we approach warm
latitudes bile and perspiration increase ; in cold latitudes they
proportionably diminish. Bichet found by experiment, that
during the first process of digestion the flow of bile is diminished, and the outlet of the stomach closed ; but as soon as
the food passes from the stomach the bile flows copiously.
With respect to the skin, the perspiration is diminished during
the preliminary process of digestion, but increases as soon as
the bile flows upon the digested food. Invalids who return
from the East or West Indies, with a diseased liver, generally
present a skin harsh and dry, with little of the moisture, or
softness of health. Whenever the skin is dry and harsh there
is an obstruction of the bile ; when it is greasy and too prone
to perspire, the bile is too abundant, and medical advice should
be taken.

Profuse perspiration of the hands and feet, particularly of
the latter, is not always to be considered as an indication of
debility ; it is often an effort of nature to throw off particles
which would be productive of disease. When it is unpleasant,
we would recommend application to a respectable practitioner,
for it is often extremely dangerous to stop it by external applications ; indeed, when profuse and acrid, it should never be
stopped except under the advice of a medical man. In slight
cases the hands and feet may be dipped in rose-water ; in bad
instances an immersion in lime-water (which is a powerful
astringent) may be more beneficial ; but, as before stated, such
applications are not safe unless directed by experience. If the
feet be dusted with powder of galls, or with alum ; or the stockings rubbed until they are saturated, with perfumed soap, and
put on when they are thoroughly dry, relief may also be obtained ; the last is however the safest application. Those who
are troubled with perspiration of the hands and feet, or with a
greasy moisture on the face, should not wear flannel next the
skin, as this will most probably increase the evil, from the close
sympathy existing between one part of the skin and the other
unless the more important considerations arising from the re-
quirements of health demand it

As the functions of the skin are so important, we will **now** give a few directions for

THE CARE OF THE SKIN.

Being assured that the preservation of health in this important membrane is one of the most effective means of prolonging life, we shall be most explicit on the subject. From what has been already said, it must be manifest, that if the pores of the skin be stopped up, the operations of digestion must be impaired, acridity and corruption of the juices must ensue, ruining the surface of the skin, and laying the foundation for acute disease. Our great object, then, is to keep the pores open by cleanliness, and give it tone by bathing and gentle friction ; and here, at the risk of being thought tautological, we shall enforce the necessity of all persons (ladies especially) passing a wet sponge over the WHOLE SURFACE of the body every morning and evening, or at any rate, every morning, commencing with tepid water, and adopting cold water as soon as they can bear it ; then let the body be thoroughly dried with a soft towel, and rubbed with a soft flesh-brush, or gently with one of Dinneford's horse-hair gloves ; the latter, at first, will not be very pleasant, but in a short time becomes a luxury. This habit will not only beautify the skin, and give it that transparency of complexion for which the Roman ladies were so eminent ; but it will be the most effectual means of guarding against colds, and all the interruptions of the system of which they are the fruitful source ; it has a double effect, it beautifies, and it fortifies the skin. The late Sir Astley Cooper has recorded, that to this habit he owed his robust health, and said that though he was in the practice of going out of hot crowded rooms at all times, night and day, without making any addition to his dress, yet he never caught a cold. It will, in fact, make woman all but divine, by removing from her everything that reminds us of mortality, leaving only that image of himself with which God has endowed her. In addition to the above practice, we also recommend bathing, whenever circumstances will permit it. We have no traces of the decline of this most invigorating custom, yet we know that it was a constant habit among the ancients. The Greek mythology represents the goddess of love rising from the sea, evidently indicating that the pure stream is the source of beauty. Lycurgus, the iron-hearted Spartan, enforced bathing by his laws, and the streams of the Eurotas daily assisted in the ablutions of the maidens of Sparta. Baths among the Greeks were among their most important public establishments, and so

imperative was the use of the baths considered, that they were
erected even on board their ships. The Romans vied with
the Greeks, nay, surpassed them, in the magnificence of their
public bathing establishments, and so moderate was the charge
for this luxury that all classes could avail themselves of it.
There are many accounts of the private and public baths of
the ancients. but we have not space for their insertion ; Sir E.
L. Bulwer has given a gorgeous description of such in his
" Last Days of Pompeii," which, doubtless, most of our readers
have perused. The French are far before us in their bathing
establishments ; in Paris there are upwards of 200 public
bathing establishments, besides those for portable baths. We
are glad that even the humblest classes will soon have such
establishments within their reach in this country.

The cold bath. does not, however, agree with all constitutions ; the person's feelings after the bath must decide its
fitness,—if it produces head-ache or excessive languor, it will
do harm : the tepid bath is, however, a most effective regenerator of the system. Dr. Armstrong gives the following nar-
ration of its advantages :—

" I consider that the advantages of tepid bathing are numerous;
and, in the first place, as a preventative of inflammatory diseases .
In many cases, the surface of the body, in this variable climate,
is chilled for some hours before the attack of external or internal inflammation ; in fact, the continuance of the chilliness is finally the cause of the inflammation, by disordering
the circulation of the blood, which, being equalized at the com-
mencement of the chilliness, by a warm bath, generally prevents
the occurrence of any acute affection of an inflammatory nature.

" In the second place, tepid bathing is extremely beneficial
in most cases of chronic rheumatism and gout, especially in
those where the functions of the stomach, liver or bowels, are
impaired.

" In the third place, it is highly beneficial in all those cases
technically and indefinitely termed wasting, or marasmus, in
children, and indigestion or dyspepsia in adults, since no single
means, in general, has more influence in restoring the natural
action of the skin, and also of those parts of the body associated in the complicated process of digestion.

" In the fourth place, it is an admirable remedy for most of
those incipient glandular affections, or ill-conditioned chronic
inflammations, which usually pass under the loose appellation
of scrofula ; and, lastly, it is so advantageous in most cutaneous
affections, that its applications to them scarcely needs a com-
ment. When we add its remarkable soothing effects in most
uterine and urinary irritations, and consider all the delightful

associations connected with perfect cleanliness, we cannot but be surprised, that tepid bathing should be so much neglected by the profession and the public of England.

"The temperature of the tepid bath should generally range between ninety-four and ninety-eight, as is most agreeable to the feeling; and it is most important *that no sense of exhaustion should be produced at the time of its use,* and no sense of *unnatural chilliness or heat immediately afterwards.* A feeling of warmth and refreshment are the certain signs of its agreeing with the patient."

It is scarcely necessary to inform my fair readers that the skin will be dried and hardened by exposure to the burning heat of the sun, or to a high wind; when such exposure is unavoidable, the face should be slightly washed by the preparation No. 24 (Appendix). On returning home, wash the face again with tepid water, and thoroughly dry it with a soft napkin. If exposed to dust or smoke, the face or neck should be wiped with a handkerchief as soon as convenient, if there be no opportunity of laving them. If sitting near the fire, persons who value their complexions must protect the face, &c., with a screen. If, from walking, or other exercise, or indeed from any cause whatever, there be moisture on the skin, a handkerchief should be applied by slight pressure, so as to absorb, not wipe it away: these are the minor cares, which, though apparently unimportant, are necessary, as their omission would destroy the appearance of the complexion.

PRECAUTIONS. A few may still be necessary. Friction to the neck and arms should be performed by means of a flesh-brush, which, though soft, is sufficiently-elastic to remove the scaly particles which sometimes appear after the application of water. When there is insufficient action in the skin, Dinneford's glove may be applied with advantage to the other parts of the body, care being taken to produce no abrasion of the skin.

All external applications are but temporary expedients, unless the stomach and intestines have their proper action. See end of Appendix, under the head of LAVEMENTS.

We shall now proceed to notice some of those appearances which are enemies to beauty.

NEVI MATERNI, or birth-marks, may be upon any part of the body, but usually appear upon the neck, face, or head; at an adult age these cannot be eradicated, but when they are observed upon an infant, the advice of a skilful surgeon should be taken. These marks are usually masses of blood-vessels, being veins when the blue color prevails, and arteries when the bright red predominates. We particularly caution mothers

against external applications to such marks, except under the advice of a surgeon.

Moles.—The common mole is situated in the middle layer of the skin ; the coloring matter is probably some chemical combination of iron ; (see Freckles ;) they are often elevated above the surface, and then the natural down of the skin over them is changed into a tuft of hair. Although they usually have their origin before birth, they sometimes appear at puberty or after life ; some also that have been observed at birth, disappear at puberty. The recipes, Nos. 21, 22, 23, 24, may be tried, (as directed in the following article, under the head of Freckles ;) if, however, they produce any irritation they must be discontinued, as dangerous consequences might ensue, if, after such warning, they were continued ; indeed, we must inform our fair readers, that the less moles are trifled with, the better, and admonish them particularly against the use of depilatories to remove the hair from them, a foetid suppurating wound is frequently the consequence of such attempts. A surgeon is the best adviser in this case.

Freckles.—These we can generally remove, by external application, but if the liver or stomach is out of order, it must have the first attention, or no external application can thoroughly succeed. Cause of Freckles.—The skin, we must inform our readers, has charcoal, or *carbon* (as the chemists term it) for its base, and in proportion as the other elements of which it is composed are driven off by heat, so will the spots upon the skin be more or less dark. Oxygen is another element of which the skin is composed, and is disengaged from carbon by heat ; if, however, iron is present, the oxygen, upon being released from the carbon, would immediately unite therewith. Now, as it is well known that there is a considerable quantity of iron in the blood, especially so in the blood of persons with red hair, the union of the oxygen with the iron will produce various shades of a rusty appearance, according to its purity and its mixture with the charcoal or carbon ; the reader will therefore at once perceive the cause of freckles, which are the rusty appearances thus produced.

Cure of Freckles.—We shall now proceed to the cure of freckles, by preparing the skin for the action of chemicals which will destroy the combination referred to, and then applying them.

For this purpose anoint the skin every night, for from three to seven days, with the Almond Paste, No. 22, or Lady Cunningham's Lip Honey, No. 21, in the Appendix ; then, if you think proper to attack the oxygen, apply the mixture No. 24 to the freckles by means of a camel-hair pencil ; persevere for

a week or ten days ; if not successful, you may be more so by
attacking the iron ; then use No. 21 or No. 22 for two or
three days, and afterwards apply No. 23, as you were directed
to do No. 24. Sometimes the freckles are so obstinate as to
resist both of these modes ; even then you may be successful,
by applying some active stimulant to the skin, which, by acting on the absorbent vessels, enables them to take up the freckles, and carry them off. No. 25 is a very excellent one,
which must be applied with a camel-hair pencil. If none of
these succeed, the Grape Lotion, No. 27, or the Lemon Cream.
No. 28, may. Remember, however, that the stomach and the
biliary system must at the same time be attended to, if they
are out of order ; for, as before said, no external applications
can eradicate those appearances effectually and permanently,
while the cause of the evil lies deeper than the skin.

YELLOW APPEARANCES sometimes present themselves under
the skin, frequently upon the neck, sometimes upon the face :
sometimes they are smaller than a sixpence, sometimes larger
than a crown. A very effectual way to remove them is, by
rubbing into them the flour of sulphur every night until they
disappear ; this, however, sometimes creates a disagreeable
odor, hence, the very frequent rubbing of the part with stone
brimstone has been adopted, and will commonly remove them
without the same disagreeable results, or No. 29 may be tried.
The mixture No. 98 may be taken at the same time, if the
stomach requires attention.

SUNBURN is nearly related to freckles, and arises from much
the same cause. No. 26 is a good preventive, and, as such.
we recommend it. When this has not been used in time to
prevent, either No. 27 or No. 28 will usually remove it.

WRINKLES.—These are still greater enemies to beauty than
the preceding, but, fortunately, are usually not seen until the
approach of old age, unless brought on by dissipation, or disease ; the latter are much the most rapid manufacturers of
wrinkles. By attention, a person with a good constitution
may prevent the exhibition of these heralds of decay for years
after the time of their common appearance ; for wrinkles are
not so certain an indication of old age, as they are of the wear
and tear of the constitution ; we, in fact, do wrong in applying the term (as generally understood) " old age," to a certain
number of years ; the approach of this period should be calculated, not by time, but by the ravages of decay. Many persons, from disease, or more often, from profligacy, are old at
thirty, while we see others of sixty with the animal spirits and
activity of matured strength. Wrinkles are occasioned by the
obstruction or obliteration of the finer blood-vessels ; when this

occurs, the larger veins are loaded, and protrude, as may be seen in the veins on the back of the hands of very aged persons; while wrinkles are in other parts produced by the absence of the blood, caused by the obstruction and obliteration above alluded to; or, by the same process acting on the small pipes which convey that moisture to the skin which keeps it smooth, soft, and flexible. Our object then is, first, to prevent wrinkles, by preserving undiminished the action of the skin, and thus securing the assistance of the minor blood-vessels; and, secondly, to direct how wrinkles may be removed if acquired. To effect the first object, we must refer to our last chapter, and we do assure our fair readers, that the system of ablution and friction there prescribed, will (unless any chronic or inflammatory disease prevents) insure them ten years' exemption from the invasion of these disagreeable reminders of mortality, beyond the period that unassisted nature would have imparted, in the present artificial state of society; observing, however, that as age advances, tepid water, instead of cold, must be used for the morning and evening ablutions. A warm bath, with friction for a quarter of an hour with a soft flesh-brush (after being thoroughly dried), will be a great regenerator of the appearance. A nutritive, but not over phlogistic diet, is also necessary to ward off these unpleasant visitors; and we need hardly say, that temperance is indispensable, and early hours equally so; for late hours will, in some degree retard our operations, or, at any rate, will prevent their proper and natural effect. The system recommended must be scrupulously followed, if wrinkles have appeared and are wished to be got rid of; in addition, No. 36 or No. 37 must be called into action, as directed in the Appendix. We need here hardly repeat, that air and exercise are also indispensable; without these, health cannot be preserved: in the absence of health, little can be done by cosmetics, except in temporary appearance.

The philosophy of the operation of destroying wrinkles is founded upon the opening, by stimulating the small thread-like blood vessels, and moisture pipes, which have been closed; if the stimulating process be pursued previous to the closing of these vessels, they will not be obliterated. Our readers will therefore perceive our directions are founded upon common sense, and that very little thought would have rendered our advice unnecessary.

CHAPTER VI.

BEAUTY OF COMPLEXION.—(*Continued.*)

PIMPLES—RINGWORM IN THE FACE—NETTLE-RASH—SMALL-POX—SCARS—
VACCINATION—WRINKLES.

No enemy to beauty, if we except the small-pox, is so effective in its destruction as pimples : these are of various kinds, some of which we shall enumerate, and give directions for their eradication. We must, however, caution our fair readers against using such nostrums as Gowland's Lotion, and even Cold Cream, (unless assured that there is in it no preparation of lead ;) indeed all repellent cosmetics are highly dangerous, as the following examples, extracted from a contemporary, will evince.

Mrs. S——, being much troubled with pimples, applied an alum poultice to her face, which was soon followed by a stroke of the palsy, and terminated in her death.   Mrs. L—— applied to her face, for pimples, a quack nostrum, supposed to be some preparation of lead.   Soon after, she was seized with epileptic fits, which ended in palsy, and caused her death.   Mr. Y—— applied a preparation of lead to his nose, to remove pimples, and it brought on palsy on one side of his face.   Miss W——, an elegant young lady of about twenty years of age, applied a cosmetic lotion to her face, to remove the "small red pimple." This produced inflammation of the liver, which it required repeated bleeding, with medicine, to remove.   As soon as the inflammation was subdued, the pimples reappeared.

The SMALL RED PIMPLE is the first we shall notice.   It is caused by obstructions of the skin, imperfect circulation, and these again arise sometimes from hereditary affection, more often from personal imprudence.   This pimple may be produced by hot rooms, violent exercise, intemperance of any kind, it also frequently appears after a foolish and dangerous, but not uncommon attempt to reduce corpulency by tne use of large doses of vinegar. Drinking cold water, eating cold vegetables, such as salads, will also, in some cases, invite these disagreeable visitants. For salads, we have, however, a great respect, and though we cannot recommend them to all, we will just say that the liberal use of oil and cayenne pepper very much assists the digestive powers in nullifying any evil which might arise from eating such viands ; obstructions and indigestion, arising from what they may, then, being the cause of these eruptions, in addition to attention to the general health, we recommend a medicated vapor bath or two, or a few warm baths will agree better with some constitutions. The Draught No. 99 being tonic, antacid, and mildly aperient, will frequently be of some assistance ; when persons have arrived at years of discretion, they can judge whether it is likely to be of service, as we have given its qualities ; but the most important of all is regular ablution and friction, air and exercise, with strict temperance, even in amusements : the search after pleasure costs many a life. For local application, Dr. Bateman's prescription, No. 29, will be found useful, particularly in removing those scaly excrescences from the skin which frequently remain when the pimples disappear. Sir Wm. Knighton's Lotion, No. 30, is a more active application. A very good lotion for the same purpose may be made by the combination of vinegar and the spirits of mindererus, (see No. 95,) or the spirit of mindererus diluted with water will sometimes prove effective, and is a very mild application.

Dr. Darwin recommends blistering the face, and cites an instance of a lady who was very much troubled with these eruptions, who, by degrees, blistered the whole of her face, and not only removed the pimples, but produced a skin more fair than she had ever previously possessed : and whenever any reappeared she at night applied the prescription No. 31. which always removed them. When, however, this ointment is used, exposure of every kind and the use of cold water had better be avoided ; the bowels also must be kept free. Mr. Plumbe, although many of his own remedies are not less violent, considers the foregoing treatment too severe, and prefers bathing the parts with warm water and gentle friction of the hand ; we think that a diluted solution of the spirit of mindererus would be still better, if the mild mode be chosen. We cannot, however, too strongly or too frequently press upon our readers that, in all these cases of pimples, attention must be paid to the stomach and bowels, and biliary system ; and that whenever a mercurial preparation is used externally or internally, all exposure to cold or damp must be avoided, and the bowels kept freely opened by mild aperients, (see No. 96,) which will agree with almost every constitution, and may be safely taken in almost every circumstance when an aperient is required.

THE WORM-PIMPLE, WITH BLACK POINTS, is one of the most common appearances, and not less unsightly than annoying. The cause of it is, obstruction of the pores of the skin, generally from want of attention ; perspiration is allowed to accumulate and become hard in the mouths of these small pipes, irritation ensues, the pimple rises, and the black point (by the vulgar supposed to be animalcula) becomes prominent. This point is, however, nothing more nor less than perspiration allowed to accumulate until it actually has the consistence of a paste, and is loaded with impurities. The only way to eradicate this appearance, when formed, is to press out the extraneous matter very carefully, and then, for a few nights apply the mild and simple application No. 22. To prevent its return, cleanliness and friction of the skin only are required, with ordinary attention to the digestive organs.

THE LIVID BUTTONY PIMPLE.—Dr. Bateman, in his work on Diseases of the skin, denominates this *Acne indurata ;* its origin is the same as the small red pimple, but it is produced in a different constitution. Attention to the state of the stomach must be the first operation for removing it. The task is, nowever, usually more tedious than with the former : we must pray our fair readers to remember, that except in extraordinary cases, there is no necessity for them to be afflicted with these excrescences ; that if they will use water and friction in the way we have so often directed, this alone will go far to prevent such appearances ; but if they will add attention to the state of the stomach, &c., &c., it is probable they never will be so troubled. We shall not go into a description of the above, its name indicates its appearance. The mode of treating it is the same as we have directed in the first case ; it may, however, be advisable to make the lotions a little stronger to facilitate the process of suppuration. Mr. Plumbe, in his work upon the Diseases of the Skin, recommends these pimples to be pricked with a needle or a lancet, to further assist the suppurative process ; when this has been affected, the matter must be squeezed out, and if any hardness or dark color remain, sponge the part frequently. Mr. Plumbe's Wash (No. 32, Appendix,) is here very useful, as is also our method of training, page 31. The Lavement, No. 91, used every other day, (for a week to ten days,) within an hour after breakfast, will also be of much service. After this. if there is any disposition to costiveness, a pint of warm water taken every day in the same manner, will generally prevent its becoming a habit

THE BARDOLPH PIMPLE; or, according to Dr. Bateman, *Acne Rosacea*, is very often rather an extensive efflorescence of the skin, than a pimple. Ladies *seldom* suffer from this frightful eruption, as it is usually caused by habits to which ladies are, we hope, never addicted—habitual potations of wine, spirits, beer! Faugh! the very enumeration of such potations in the same page that the sex is mentioned, is almost an insult to it; but lest some unfortunate should have imbibed such habits we will proceed to advise as to its extirpation; first premising, that indulgence of the appetite by the immoderate use of highly seasoned dishes will also favor this appearance. The Bardolph eruption is characterized by a collection of small suppurating pimples, accompanied with a shining redness and an irregular bumpy appearance of that portion of the face which is affected; the nose usually receives its first assaults, and from thence the disease spreads over a large portion of the face, until in process of time a frightful network of veins, with small red lines stretching across the cheeks, give the face that frightful appearance which so pointedly marks the habitual sot and sensualist. At this stage it is seldom cured. In the earlier periods, a careful examination would usually reveal small collections of matter deeply seated under the red appearances. This matter should be let out with a needle or the point of a lancet, swelling and redness would then disappear; warm water, fomentations, and friction with a soft brush, must then be persevered in, and if the habits be reformed, the stomach attended to as before advised, and our mode of training adopted, even this dreadful destroyer of beauty may be conquered. But all highly seasoned meats, cold vegetables, mustard, cayenne, strong liquors, pickles, &c., must be absolutely avoided.

NETTLE-RASH.—From the terms used one would almost be tempted to suppose our physicians wished to disguise these eruptions under the prettiness of the names with which they have distinguished them. *Roseola* is the medical term for this rash. This affection is caused by acidity and general disorder of the stomach; the viands most likely to produce it, if used immoderately, are lobsters, crabs, shrimps, oysters, most shellfish, pork, mushrooms, stone-fruit of all kinds, green cucumber, vinegar. The eruption has been designated more ludicrous than dangerous. It is, however, very unpleasant. The appearance is very common, and often not suspected to be the above disease. It presents a series of roseate colored patches, frequently with a swelling, with a hard border, of a paler color than the rash in the centre of the patches; and it is accompanied, sometimes by an itching, sometimes a tingling, sensation.

3

The bowels must be freely opened; two spoonsful of the draught No. 97, taken three times a day for a week, will generally remove it. Ladies, however, must again be reminded that the uterine system must not be forgotten in all cases where aperients are recommended. The medicine may be assisted by *slightly* sponging the face occasionally with a weak solution of tepid rain water.

TETTER, *or Ring-worm of the Face.*—The former is the more expressive name; it is totally different from the ring-worm of the head, and, like the eruptions already noticed, is occasioned by a disordered stomach, which, vitiating the blood, and deranging the functions of the skin, causes these disagreeable humors. This fact, no doubt, originated a common expression, " Better out than in ;" so it is, but the cause for its being *in* must be removed ; and then, in the early stage, we have no objection to facilitate its disappearance by the application of Eau de Cologne in the following proportion : one pint of water, four pints of Eau de Cologne ; or, the lotion No. 33, (Appendix.) The parts may be frequently sponged with either of these, the bowels being properly attended to by mild aperients, assisted occasionally with the lavements as before directed ; there are several given in the Appendix, some stronger than the others ; these are easily distinguished by the reader, and must be adopted as experience may have directed. Be it, however, specially remembered, that no repellent applications must be used when the blisters of the eruption once appear ; the above external application must only be adopted at the earliest stage, when the stiffness of the parts has given warning of the approaching tetter. When the disease has taken hold of the constitution, we should generally recommend medical advice ; it may, however, even then, in ordinary cases, be removed without it, but with us the safest plan is best. To enable our readers to distinguish it, and to apply proper remedies, at *the proper time*, we shall describe its *cause* and appearance.

It usually, as before stated, arises from a disordered stomach, and, in addition, the suppression of perspiration ; colds, particularly when chilliness of the skin has been remarkable, sore throats, and even fatigue from over-exertion, are frequently followed by this eruption. Obstructions of the uterine system, also piles, are sometimes the occasion of its appearance. The symptoms by which we are premonished of the disease, are slight shiverings, flushes of the face, headache, pains in the limbs, stiffness and itching, or tingling of the parts where the ring-worm will appear, and sometimes a considerable accession of fever. The affected part then becomes red, little blisters appear (we must NOT, when this stage is arrived, attempt to drive them in) in clusters, frequently at the corners of the mouth, or on the edges of the lips; sometimes they form a circle round the mouth, from whence the term *ringworm* was doubtless adopted; the nose, and sometimes the chin, is the seat of the disease. These blisters are filled with a transparent fluid, which, in about twenty-four hours, becomes turbid and of a yellowish white, which is succeeded by a brown yellow matter; the lips, or other parts affected, become hard and swollen, with a sensation of heat and smarting,— this, in three or four days, is relieved by the escape of the matter, which forms thick dark crusts. This must NOT be picked off; for if let alone, the swelling will subside, and in four or five days these crusts will fall off; if, however, they are removed by violence, other matter will be formed, and the parts become again encrusted; *if, however,* EACH BLISTER be carefully pricked with a needle, and the fluid pressed out *before it becomes turbid and milky,* much pain will be prevented, and the irritation will sooner subside. The entire course of the disease usually occupies about ten or twelve days.

CURE.—Two spoonsful of the draught No. 97 may be taken three times a day; if too exciting or weakening, No. 99 may be adopted after a day or two; the first is generally the best. Or the bowels, if tolerably regular, may be kept open by either of the lavements which are found to agree. When the eruption becomes painful, or itches violently, the sedative lotion, No. 34, may be often applied by means of a sponge gently drawn over it; if this is found too strong, a little more water may be added. Our system of training, modified by circumstances, will here again be of great service. During all these eruptions, malt liquors must be avoided. After the disappearance of the blister, the pill No. 94 may be taken every other day for a week; it will much assist in cleansing the system.

ON SCARS.—Without commencing another chapter, we will say a few words upon scars. They may be caused by accident or disease, but are equally enemies to beauty.

Since the introduction of vaccination, the scars arising from the latter are confined almost to boils, or tumors of a more serious nature. We will, however, enable our readers to judge if vaccination has been effectually performed by stating the ordinary process, the appearances which ought to be exhibited, and a test or two of effective vaccination.

1st.—The matter should be taken from a subject upon the ninth day, and inserted under the skin of the patient.

2nd.—On the third day afterwards, a small red spot should appear.

3d.—On the sixth day it should become discolored in the centre.

4th.—On the tenth day it is surrounded with inflammation, and should have a dimple in the centre, and not be raised like an ordinary pimple.

5th.—It should disappear about the thirteenth day, and the scales should fall off in about a fortnight.

Take notice that the shape of the pustule is *oval* or *circular*, the margin of it should be even, *not* jagged, and the outer part of a deeper red than the space within it.

Tests.—On the 5th day, vaccinate the second arm from matter taken from the first ; if the virus has been effective, both pustules will ripen on the same day ; if this does not take place, the constitution has not been properly affected, and the operation must be repeated, either at once or within some short space of time. This is called Dr. Bryer's test.

Dr. Gregory has stated, (and his statement is borne out by experience,) that when the scar left upon the arm is distinct, circular, and full of little pits or dimples, spreading, as it were, in rays from a centre, and the scar is so small as to be covered with a *pea*, that then, if secondary small-pox do occur, it will be so slight as neither to affect the complexion nor the constitution ; but on the contrary, if the scar be large, irregular, without the radiated pits, it is probable, if the patient is ever affected with small-pox, that it will be severe ; the patient should therefore, in the latter case, be again operated upon. As the virus will not take effect if the scar be perfect, the process should be repeated if the parent has any doubt upon the subject. This is termed Dr. Gregory's test.

Another test is sometimes adopted upon the fifth day, viz., prick the vesicle with a needle ; if it be a genuine vaccine pustule, the whole of the contents will not be evacuated, for this reason, that the pustule is composed of a series of small cells that do not communicate the one with the other, while the ordinary pimple has but one cell.

Caution.—If ever secondary small-pox should occur, care must be taken not to break the pustules, nor rub off the incrustation, or pitting will occur. To allay their irritation or itching, take a small portion of cream, mixed with a little pure chalk, or magnesia : apply it with a camel's hair pencil.

It has been said that the efficacy of vaccination is not permanent—that it loses its virtue in the course of ten or fifteen years : such is not always the case ; but there are many *well-established* cases of the virtue being lost in seven. Let those, then, who are under the apprehension, repeat the operation within that time, and they will be safe ; at any rate from any injurious result as to personal appearance or to health, even if they should take it. We shall now proceed to

SCARS FROM TUMORS.—The late Sir Astley Cooper has left upon record the following advice to young surgeons. It is very interesting.

" The prevention of scars is a great object, particularly in exposed parts of the body. This may appear of little consequence, but it certainly is not so. Scars from abscesses in the necks of females excite in the minds of most of our sex a reluctance to associate with them ; and thus many a fine young woman may, by such scars, be doomed to perpetual celibacy. No part of the practice of surgery has been more faulty, than the manner in which abscesses of the neck have been treated. I have seen, on one side of the neck, large scars from abscesses that have been badly managed ; whilst, on the other side, where the treatment had been more skilful, scarcely any vestige of a wound was to be seen.

" I have from very early practice, and subsequent experience has proved to me its use, been exceedingly careful in the management of these cases.

" Aperients, with calomel and rhubarb, should be given, and evaporating lotions should be used ; you must be strict as to regimen and diet ; the food must be nutritive, but not stimulating. The best mode to adopt is to open the abscess before the skin be much affected, and as soon as a blush has appeared ; thus scars will in general be prevented. One more observation is of the highest importance. Let me entreat you not to open these tumors when they have a purple blush upon them like the hue of a grape ; the skin is then thin, and the wound will slough ; and if you then open the tumor, you will bring disgrace upon yourself. When you press the sides of the wound, take care to squeeze out all the solid flakes of matter to be met with in scrofulous tumors. If this be not attended to, they will at last slough ; but if, on the contrary, you carefully avoid leaving any of that unorganized substance, adhesion will take place, and the wound will heal. Almost everything in these cases depends on getting rid of the solid matter. Bread poultices, made with a solution of sulphate of zinc and spirits, may be afterwards used."

SCARS FROM ACCIDENTS.—" In burns and scalds the skin is apt to be drawn together in folds, and have a disagreeable mixture of marks, some too red, and some too white. The best method of preventing this is by healing the sore as speedily as possible ; and when any unsightly excrescence is observed to be forming on the scar, to reduce it by caustic."

When a cut from glass or a knife occurs, the simplest mode

to prevent a permanent scar, is, to draw the edges of the wound close together, being careful that no foreign matter remains within, then bind them firmly with strips of diachylon plaster. A recipe for a very good court plaster will be found at No. 35, Appendix, which may be used for trifling cuts or excoriations.

Let it, however, be remembered, that in severe cuts or contused wounds, a surgeon should always be sent for, and more especially if a scar is wished to be avoided

CHAPTER VII.

BEAUTY OF THE ARMS, HANDS, AND FEET.

COLOR OF THE HANDS—WASHING AND DRYING THE HANDS—FRICTION OF
THE HANDS—SOAPS—GLOVES—SLEEPING IN GLOVES—THE NAILS—CARE
OF—CHAPS—CHILBLAINS—WARTS—REMEDIES FOR THEM—TIGHT SHOES
—CORNS—PRESERVATION OF THE FEET.

THE study of the anatomical structure of the human body is
eminently calculated to impart elevated ideas of the great
Being who has, by such extraordinary contrivances, imparted
to it strength united with beauty. The structure of the arms,
hands, and feet, exhibits wonderful instances of this association,
and we much regret that our space prevents us from describ-
ing it. We are confined, then, to the details of the best way of
ensuring to the hands, feet, &c., the greatest degree of beauty
of which they are susceptible.

The directions we have already given respecting the skin
and complexion are particularly applicable to improving the
appearance of the arms. Let the arms be washed in lukewarm water, thoroughly dried, and then well rubbed with a
soft brush, or lightly with a hair glove ; this will assist in producing that roundness which is so desirable. To produce
whiteness, the arm must constantly be covered ; at night,
wash, &c., as before directed ; then rub the arms with the unguent No. 58 ; put on white kid gloves : repeat this for a
week, and it will produce a softness almost magical ; that is,
in ordinary cases ; in some it must be continued for a longer
period : the hands will of course be included in the operation,
and no chaps or chilblains will ever appear while the practice
is continued, unless from persisting in holding the hands to the
fire when damp, or when just coming out of the cold air. The
process above recommended will usually ensure softness and
whiteness of the hand ; the latter must, however, of course in
some measure depend upon the natural complexion. Habits

will also have a great effect in facilitating or retarding our object ; the less the hand is used or exposed, the softer and whiter it is likely to become : if the employment is such as tends to incornute the hand, softness cannot be obtained ; but to such employments, ladies are seldom obnoxious. For merely whitening the hands, the recipes 83 and 84 are perhaps even more efficacious than No. 58.

CHILBLAINS, CHAPS.—Exposure to severe cold, followed by close approximation to the fire, will usually produce chilblains. They are also occasioned by an imperfect circulation of the blood : everything, therefore, that causes the circulation to be regular, tends to prevent chilblains. Persons who are liable to them should be very particular in thoroughly drying the hands and feet ; every morning and evening, as winter approaches, they should wash the feet in lukewarm water, or, what would be much better, in the solution No. 64, dry them thoroughly, and then rub the feet and legs with a hair glove for ten minutes or a quarter of an hour : such persons ought never to go near a fire for some time after they come out of the external air ; let them, instead, have the feet and hands well rubbed ; warmth will be communicated quicker by this process than by fire, and the general health will be improved. If, in spite of these precautions, any symptoms of chilblains appear, anointing the feet night and morning, after washing, with the unguent No. 63 (Appendix), will in ordinary cases prevent their appearance. If chilblains have appeared, the lotion No. 59, with friction of the legs and feet, when it can be borne, and attention to our general remarks, will remove them.

We cannot too strongly impress upon our readers the fact, that chilblain is an ARTIFICIAL MALADY, produced generally by the sudden application of heat to parts which are extremely cold ; it usually appears upon the hands and feet, first, from the imperfect circulation of the blood at such extremities ; and second, from their being more liable to be exposed to the fire on ordinary occasions. Let it be remembered that cold draughts of air admitted into hot rooms are frequent sources of chilblains, when they come in immediate contact with the extremities. Sitting over a fire with the feet upon the fender, ought, then, to be avoided ; and in large parties keep as far from the door as conveniently can be done.

CHAPS.—If our readers will use the unguent No. 58, and pay attention to our directions, we will guarantee them from chapped hands ; therefore we shall say no more upon the subject, but proceed at once to another cause of injury to the beauty of the hand, viz. :

WARTS, which are a great disfigurement to the hand, may

be always removed by perseverance: if applied night and morning on their first appearance, common ink will remove them. When they have been clearly developed, a certain means of extirpating them is the following: Take a small piece of court-plaster made upon india-rubber webbing, cut a hole in its centre just sufficiently large to admit the head of the wart, rub this head with lunar caustic night and morning; when it becomes hard, pick off the top, and again apply the caustic; the solution No. 56, in the Appendix, applied with a camel's hair brush, is more convenient. The use of the court-plaster is to prevent the surrounding skin from being injured; it is therefore of much importance, as severe wounds are sometimes made when it is absent. Be very careful in applying the solution, as it will destroy the clothes—wash the camel's hair brush each time it is used, or it will quickly be destroyed. The tincture No. 57 will also frequently be effective in its operations, as also will No. 56: this is usually successful, but we prefer either of the others. Whenever a caustic solution is used, the top of the wart must be picked off as often as it becomes hard: if this plan be pursued, the warts will, by one or the other of the above preparations, be generally removed within a month, often within ten days. Sometimes they are very tiresome: in such cases, when one remedy does not make a visible progress towards extirpating them, try another. Apply all these mixtures with a camel's hair pencil. The liquid from the application No. 60 is also very effective; it must be allowed to dry on; the oftener it is applied the better.

The feet are exposed to excrescences even more painful than warts upon the hand. These are generally produced by tight shoes; we fear, however, that our fair friends will wear such so long as little feet are considered pretty; we shall, therefore, not waste words by advising them to the contrary.

Corns.—If our readers will recollect that the shape of the corn is that of an inverted cone, consequently, that pressure upon it must force the point further into the flesh, they will not wonder at the dreadful pain occasioned by wearing tight shoes when they have acquired corns; as long as this is persisted in, the corn will increase in size, for the inflammation caused by this pressure continually adds to the corn. The same idea, however, suggests a remedy; for if pressure be removed from the excrescence it will in time disappear. A mode of making this description of corn plaster will be found at No. 62, of the Appendix. No. 61 is said to be an infallible corn plaster, and we have seen many instances of the success-

3*

With respect to the beauty of the eye, we may remark, that a large pupil is now, and always has been, considered a beauty. Homer speaks of the ox-eyed Juno, and all allow the beauty of the gazelle-eyed Leila, as described by Byron :—

> "Her eye's dark charm 't were vain to tell,
> But gaze on that of the gazelle,
> It will assist thy fancy well ;
> As large, as languishingly dark,
> But soul beam'd forth in every spark
> That darted from beneath the lid
> Bright as the jewel of Giamschid.
> Yea, soul ! and should our prophet say
> That form was nought but breathing clay,
> By Alla, I would answer nay,
> Though on Al Sirat's arch I stood,
> Which totters o'er the fiery flood."

A large pupil is, then, esteemed beautiful ; but it is scarce-ly to be desired, as it is usually an indication of a weakly constitution, and is most common with persons of consumptive habits.

The most important object we have in view at present is the preservation of the eye : to this end, we must press our read-to abandon the use of all kinds of glasses, unless they are absolutely and imperatively obliged to use them. Preserving glasses are just names for certain machines which should be called sight-destroyers ; for when these are once adopted, the magnifying spectacles will soon be necessary. Green spectacles are even worse than the light ones termed preservers. If the eye is weak, nine times out of ten, cold pump water is the best lotion. Strengthening lotions, when composed of spirits or acids, are stimulants : such, of course, must occasionally be used, but judgment is required in using them, and a surgeon's direction is generally required when these become necessary. Sometimes, when the eye is inflamed, it will be relieved by a lotion made of one teaspoonful of good brandy in a wineglass-ful of water ; but as inflammation may arise from different causes, sometimes requiring anodynes, sometimes stimulants, we can only give such, and leave the use of them to the judgment of the reader. (See Appendix, Nos. 46, 47.)

If the eyes are inclined to be inflamed after being up late, the unguent No. 45, rubbed on both lids when retiring to rest, will generally almost magically relieve them. Nine times out of ten, supposed affections of the eye are only inflammations of the eye-lid : in such cases this unguent will effect a cure. If in the evening the eye should be inflamed, wash it carefully with warm water, dry it thoroughly, and an hour afterwards apply the lotion No. 46, which is an excellent remedy when the ball of the eye has a prickly sensation, as though sand were in it. Experience will teach which sort of collyrium is required ; but as the eye is a delicate organ, we cannot advise that it should be trifled with.

SQUINTING.—Science has now discovered an operation that will effectually cure squinting. It is not either painful or dangerous ; but we strongly advise none to submit to it until they have arrived at the age of from nineteen to twenty-one, as, if it be done before, it is more than probable that the eye will be drawn the contrary way by the time they reach that age. A more simple remedy is to cover the stronger eye, which will compel the weaker one to exertion, and thus increase its power. Perseverance in this plan is generally successful.

Our fair friends often injure the eye by wearing white veils The glitter which this causes, and the constant exercise to which its continual shifting exposes the eye in following its movements, is often the occasion of great injury to the sight.

The LIPS now demand our attention. It is hardly necessary to remark, that the fresh ruby-colored lips, so highly praised by the poets, is the sign of health. Those who attend to our previous observations under the head of TRAINING, may almost ensure them. When the health is impaired, the lips can only have an artificial redness. Some of our fair readers, enjoying good health, and conscious of possessing ruby lips, may, however, be annoyed by their chapping : the Appendix furnishes an excellent remedy, No. 51 ; and an excellent preventive, No. 21. An early attention to the latter will prevent this distressing affliction.

From the lips we very readily transfer our remarks to the BREATH. Its purity is of the greatest consequence ; what, indeed, could be so afflicting to one of the gentle sex as impurity in this respect? yet it may occur without any neglect on her part, and, we are sorry to say, it is not always that a remedy can be offered ; in other words, there are cases where it is incurable.

One great cause of this affliction is the existence of a superabundance of phosphate of lime in the fluids of the mouth, which leaves a deposit upon the teeth, familiarly known by the term *tartar :* this has a particularly unpleasant effluvium ; and when once deposited, favors the lodgment of small particles of food ; and these, if not removed, decompose, become incorporated with the tartar, and produce a most abominable odor, which is taken up by the breath as it passes out of the mouth. This, probably, is the occasion of fetid breath in ninety-nine cases out of every hundred. We have already stated that it is much easier to assign a reason for this affliction than it is to relieve it ; but we must confess that even this poor satisfaction is not always afforded us, so secret are some of the operations of nature.

MODE OF PROCEDURE TO CURE FETID BREATH.—Let the teeth be well examined ; let those which are hollow or broken be removed or stopped ; and remember it is useless to go to the advertising quack-doctors. They will stop teeth, and draw teeth, and put in teeth ; but in the first and last case it is probable that the effluvium will be increased, and in the second case, you MAY *haply* escape without your jaw being broken ; if so, be very thankful ; but go to a man of standing and station in his profession.

The teeth having been examined and set to rights, our next advice is to keep them so by always brushing them, after eating, with or without tooth-powder. There are several excellent dentrifices in the Appendix : No. 39 or 40 would be beneficial in this case ; perhaps the latter might be the best. It must not, however be forgotten that cleansing the teeth does not remove the cause of the tartar, viz., the superabundance of phosphate of lime in the saliva. For this purpose the draughts No. 53 and 54 are admirably adapted. No. 55 is stronger than 54, and may be substituted if the state of the stomach warrants it : both are tonic and aperient. Whenever we speak of constitutional affections, we must remind the reader of our directions as to diet and habits : if these are attended to, they will much assist in removing all disarrangements of the system.

For further information respecting the teeth, see next chapter.

CHAPTER IX.

BEAUTY OF THE TEETH, GUMS, ETC.

THE title of this chapter at once suggests the importance of the preservation of these invaluable organs. A good set of teeth is one of the most remarkable ornaments of the " human face divine." It produces a pleasurable feeling in the beholder, and, as it were, prepares him favorably for an introduction : it also preserves to the features their natural symmetry : when the teeth decay, this is destroyed.' When the side teeth are removed, the alveolar process becomes absorbed, the cheeks fall in, and age becomes prematurely stamped upon the countenance. If the front teeth are absent, the appearance of premature old age is even more strongly and more quickly exhibited, from the lips losing their only support. As forming one of the organs of articulation, the teeth are equally important ; but the most important office is, undoubtedly, the mastication of the food, and the preparation of it for the digestive powers of the stomach. Attention, then, to the preservation of the teeth cannot be commenced too early. In their daily ablutions, children should be taught always to include their teeth : nor can parents commence too early attending to their children's teeth ; by it irregularity may be prevented, and a fine set of teeth insured in ninety-nine cases out of a hundred, that is, if the attention be accompanied by judicious measures. Five dollars paid to a first-rate dentist for advice respecting a child's teeth, when malformation or disarrangement is first seen, would generally pay the parent abundant interest for the outlay. But our space will not permit us to enlarge upon this point further than to warn parents against habitual use of Grey powders, blue powders, calomel, blue pill, or mercury in any form.

These must occasionally be resorted to by medical men ; but their indiscriminate use by unprofessional persons is destructive not only to teeth, but the constitution.   To the use of mercury in their childhood, very many persons unconsciously owe the early decay of their teeth.

Let it be also remembered that the character of a child's food has much influence upon the teeth.   Simple food will not generate tartar, while all heated food, spices, acids, or saccharine compositions, (let them be called *bon-bons*, or by any other fashionable and foolish terms,) will disorder the stomach, and create a disposition in the saliva to deposit tartar.   They will also cause tooth-ache, and the little sufferer then endures the torture which should only arise from natural decay or matured indulgence in sensual gratification ; inflicted, be it recollected, by the hands which ought to have sheltered it from harm.   The mischief does not, however, end with the pain ; in after life all the mortification arising from having a bad set of teeth, will, in very numerous instances, be attributed to the negligence or the weakness of the parent.

When a child reaches the age of six, or from that to eight years, it begins to lose the first teeth, and to obtain the permanent teeth.   This is the most important time ; attention should then be directed to the appearance of the second set, and a dentist ought occasionally to examine the child's mouth, which, as we have before said, amply repays the parent for the trouble and expense.   Sometimes the temporary teeth require removing, to allow the permanent ones to take their proper place ; and if this be neglected at the proper time, a lasting deformity is produced, which can only be remedied by severe pain ; *i. e.*, the removal of those which have been found out of their place, and the substitution of artificial teeth.   Need we say more to force this necessity upon the attention of MOTHERS ?

In the preceding chapter we have directed the attention of grown persons to the necessity of having their teeth examined by a dentist, under certain circumstances.   The dentist, be it recollected, in what is termed scaling the teeth, does not remove any portion of them, but merely the *caries*, which have fixed themselves, like a cement, upon them.   To such an extent is this accumulation, that many persons have never even seen their teeth, probably, from the age of childhood.   The filthiness of this practice is thus alluded to by Dr. Bell, the celebrated anatomical lecturer :—

" When the disgusting effects of this accumulation are considered, it would appear impossible that any persuasion could be necessary to induce persons to obviate so great a nuisance, even on their own account ; or, if they are too debased to procure their own comfort and cleanliness at the expense of a very little care and trouble, they surely have no right to shock the senses of others who possess more delicacy and propriety of feeling than themselves. Yet so it is; and the sight and the smell are alike constantly outraged by the filthiness of people who seem to obtrude their faces the closer in proportion to the disgust which they occasion."

The teeth having been attended to, may easily be kept in proper order by ordinary attention, that is to say, may usually be so kept: constitutional derangement will, of course, destroy them; and here the habits before recommended by us force themselves upon our attention. If the whole system of training is not pursued, let us press the necessity of the ablutions and friction: these assist the constitution almost miraculously. TOOTH-BRUSHES should not be too hard; indeed, a soft one is best: we know none better than those formed of the root of marsh-mallows, designated vegetable tooth-brushes, which are thus described by a veteran perfumer. We give HIS OWN WORDS, with all his cautions.

"Take marine marsh-mallows roots, (so called from growing in salt water marshes;) cut them into lengths of five or six inches, and of the thickness of a middling rattan cane. Dry them pretty well in the shade, but not so much as to make them shrivel. Now pulverize, finely, two ounces of good dragon's-blood, and put it into a flat-bottomed glazed pan, with four ounces of highly rectified spirit, and half an ounce of fresh conserve of roses. Set the pan over a gentle charcoal fire, and keep stirring it until all the gum (dragon's blood) is dissolved; then put in about thirty or forty of the marsh-mallow sticks; stir them about with a knife, and carefully turn them, so that all parts may absorb the dye alike. Do this until the bottom of the pan be quite dry, from absorption and evaporation of the spirit; but still keep shaking and stirring over the decaying fire, until the sticks or roots are perfectly dry and hard."

REMARKS.—"Both ends of each root or stick, should, previous to immersion in the pan, be bruised gently by a hammer, for half an inch downwards, so as to open its fibres, and thereby form a brush."

Further Remarks.—"These sticks or brushes are generally used by dipping one of the ends in a powder or opiate, (see Appendix from No. 38,) and then by rubbing them against the teeth, which they cleanse and whiten in a most admirable manner; indeed, better than by anything else ever invented.'

Additional Remarks.—" The genuine is easily known from
the spurious kind by the shade of color ; the former being
bright red or scarlet, whilst the latter are merely purple. The
former cleanse the teeth from the gum contained in them :
whilst the latter do so merely by friction."

Some persons, however, do not like these vegetable brushes ;
such, then, should obtain a tooth-brush moderately soft, and
cleanse the teeth morning and evening with one of the dentifrices in the Appendix; (see No. 38.) the brush having been
dipped in lukewarm water. Neither hot nor cold water should
ever be used to the teeth : severe and permanent tooth-ache is
frequently brought on by sudden changes of their temperature.
It is well ascertained that teeth possess vitality, though not of
a very active kind ; and thus the shock produced by the sudden application of cold or hot water may produce a degree of
inflammation, which will only subside from the removal of the
tooth which has been the particular seat of the excitement.
In the Appendix we have given several washes for the teeth ;
and to enable the reader to choose such, (or a dentifrice,) we
have usually designated them by their qualities, rather than by
names without meaning. One of these, as above noticed,
should be used night and morning, first brushing upwards and
downwards, then across, and lastly repeating the first operation. This simple process requires care ; the first process
particularly should be performed without violence, or the gum
will, to a certain extent, be gradually pushed from its propei
place on the teeth. Those persons who have any defect in the
teeth or breath, should use the tooth-brush after every meal :
it were better that all should do so ; tooth-picks would then be
unnecessary. These instruments are very dangerous ; those
formed of gold, silver, or any metal, should never be used
when one is necessary ; a quill is the best material of which
it can be made. The tooth-powders we have given may be
used without danger ; but we must caution our readers against
using advertised dentifrices, of the composition of which they
know nothing. Many of them do produce for a time a beautiful appearance, which is, however, usually succeeded by perma
nent injury : acid of some sort, is in them, the most operative
ingredient, which certainly cleanses the teeth, but in time must
destroy the enamel.

TOOTH-ACHE

now claims our attention. We cannot too seriously press
upon the attention of our fair readers the fact, that if they have
frequent tooth-ache, the probability is that the seat of the dis-

order is in the stomach. If so, and it be not attended to, they may torture themselves with stimulating local applications, but we can assure them that these can only give temporary relief, (not always even that,) and probably at the expense of destroying the appearance of the teeth.

In any serious attack of tooth-ache, then, we recommend our readers to take a few aperient draughts or pills; No. 94, every other morning for a week, will be very beneficial; after which, the draught No. 98 may be taken to assist in removing the mercury from the system : or No. 98 may be first tried, and if not effective, the former mode adopted. If the system be debilitated, united with irregularity of the digestive organs, one of those numbered 54 or 97 may be better still ; but in any complicated disarrangement of the system, medical advice will be the best, and, indeed, the most economical. For local application, see Nos. 87 to 89. If these fail, No. 90 is an excellent fomentation to allay the pains while the medicine is acting on the system : in addition, put both the feet in warm water, going to bed ; and if this procedure does not take effect in a day or two, the tooth must be stopped or taken out. The gums may, however, be in such a state of inflammation that this operation would be dangerous : a respectable dentist would be the best judge of this. When you go to him, be sure to inform him what means you have taken to obtain relief. Mr. Saunders, to whose book we have before alluded, is, like ourselves, well assured that tooth-ache very frequently arises from indigestion, and is frequently, therefore, cured by a judicious use of tonic and aperient medicines. He advises the use of the pill No. 100, as described, used alternately with those numbered 101. In such case the draught given on page 31 may be very beneficial, especially when aloes does not agree with the person. As this malady frequently arises from cold, we cannot too strenuously urge the necessity of keeping the feet DRY and WARM. Damp and cold feet are a frequent cause not only of tooth-ache, but of very many inflammatory diseases.

CHAPTER X.

BEAUTY OF THE HAIR.

STRUCTURE OF THE HAIR—RULES FOR THICKENING AND DYEING THE HAIR—GENERAL MANAGEMENT OF THE HAIR—OILS—WASHES—PERFUMERY.

THE hair has ever been considered one of the most beautiful ornaments of women ; its beauty is not confined to color ; although in our times red hair is banished from the catalogue of the graces, the painters and poets of former days have immortalized those "golden locks ;" the pictures of our best masters have been remarkably distinguished in this respect. A hint has just been given us, that this color is most manageable in a picture ; and a cynic at our elbow would insinuate that this was the reason of the preference of the ancient masters ; also, that we are equally wrong in assuming that the poets patronized them ; for auburn, not red, hair was distinguished by the epithet "golden." We must leave the discussion to be settled by the casuists, for we have not space for the controversy ; nor would our conscience permit us to allow the beautiful faces we have seen thus shadowed, to be deprived of their smiles, by the record of a sentence of excommunication pronounced against the ornaments of their heads.

The diversified arrangement of the hair will give almost as many changes to the expression of the face as there may be changes in the form of the hair ; when, therefore, this is of luxuriant growth, it is justly and most highly esteemed by the possessor, the arrangement alone making up for the deficiency of beauty in the features.

The natural parting of the hair in the front of the head is highly esteemed when it proceeds in a straight line from the crown of the head to the forehead, as the eye of the beholder is, as it were, carried forward by the line presented by the nose : an appearance which all admire, though perhaps unconscious of the cause of their pleasure. The heads of Raphael, Correggio, and Guido, present admirable illustrations of this beauty, which, therefore, was evidently highly valued by the old masters. Heads which have this peculiarity are usually characterized by great developments of the cerebrum; and, according to physiognomists, such heads usually indicate that the individual habitually possesses elevated ideas and strong mental powers. The works of the ancients seem to argue that this is no new idea, as that appearance of the head is very generally adopted by them. We do not vouch for the fact, although we are inclined to believe that the parting alluded to, is generally found in heads where the mental part of the cranium is large and high.

Before we proceed to give directions for beautifying the hair, we shall give M. Chevalier's anatomical sketch of it, as given in a work published in 1825, and now but little known. We could give reasons for doubting some portions of his statement, but it is sufficiently accurate for our present purpose, and he is a respectable authority.

" Both the long hairs and the pubescence, or down, which consists of an infinite number of minute hairs, have this in common, that they grow from small bulbs imbedded in the surface of the inner or true skin, where they are supplied by vessels from a net-like tissue appropriated for their nourishment From the outer surface of the true skin they pass through the membrane of color and the scarf skin, at very acute angles, closely embraced by both, especially by the latter, which sheathes their protrusion so firmly as not to allow them easily to be detached, even after a length of maceration and putrefaction which has been sufficient to destroy the membrane of color, so that, in this respect, the hair resembles the nails. It is evident, from this arrangement, that the capillary perforations or pores through which the hairs pass, cannot be perspiratory; for the obliquity of their course, and their firm adhesions, would oppose a serious, if not an insurmountable obstacle to the transmission of anything through them, while they are in a natural state. It must constitute a perfectly valvular obstruction. The hairs are inserted, or, perhaps, we should rather say, rooted, on the exterior part of the true skin, in such a manner, as, together with this obliquity of their direction, to make them astonishingly secure in their allotted situations. In a great number of animals they appear to be like slender horns, conical in their form, and, as it were, hermetically closed at the point, and are periodically shut off. In the sheep, they continue to grow, that they may be sheared for the benefit of their purveyors and protectors. For wool is hair

adapted to particular circumstances ; and we know that change
of climate will, in some instances, cause a change from the
one form of growth to the other, so as to fit the animal for its
new residence. In man, they are tubular ; and the tubes are
intersected by partitions, resembling, in some degrees, the sap
vessels of plants ; such, for instance, as are beautifully seen in
slitting up the leaves and stalks of the bur-reed, called by bot-
anists, *Spurganium ramosum*, and other aquatic plants, which
shoot up in the marshes their beautiful but obtrusive and de-
ceitful verdure. The hairs being intended for protection from
violence, as well as for covering, they are thus formed on the
same principle as the bones themselves ; their hollowness pro-
venting incumbrance from their weight, with rather an increase than a diminution of their powers of resistance, on account of the rounded form of their transverse sections.
"Whether the hairs transmit any secretion, may be worthy
of inquiry. That those of the head have a peculiar odor,
which is often retained for many years after their separation
from it, is well known ; and we have cases on record, in which
the removal of them from the head at an early period after
acute diseases, has been followed by alarming symptoms,
scarcely to be accounted for by the mere additional exposure
to cold. But, at all events, when the extent of the whole system of the hair is considered, it will be found to bear no incon-
siderable or unimportant proportion in the animal economy ;
and it will necessarily follow, that those diseases of the skin,
which extend deep enough to destroy their originations, must,
on this very account, even if that were all, expose the whole
frame to some serious derangements. If the morbid state of
one gland, as that of the breast, or an absorbent gland, shall
affect the whole constitution with disease, these parts, so
countless in numbers and essential in function, may be natural-
ly expected to have an influence of large, though, perhaps, not
immediately perceptible amount on the general health of the
body, making up, by their numbers, for the smallness of their
size, in the share which they, and the pores into which they
are inserted, take in the balance of the constitutional actions.
"It must be further observed, respecting the pubescence or
down of the skin, that the hairs composing it pass from the
inner skin to the surface of the body in pairs or triplets, per-
forating the net-like vessels, and both the membrane of color
and the scarf skin, at very acute angles ; so that by the form
of their bulbous insertions, and the direction in which they
proceed outward, they serve to connect together all the parts
of the skin, like so many fine pins or fastenings, adding to the
entireness and security of the whole system. "

Methods of beautifying the Hair.—We need hardly in form our readers that with respect to the hair particular cleanliness is absolutely necessary : it must be thoroughly brushed and combed every morning and evening ; the brush should also be brought into requisition at each time of dressing, or the dust will accumulate upon the long hair of ladies.

In the Appendix we have given a number of recipes for hair oils, washes, dyes, depilatories, perfumed waters, and *esprits.* These receipts produce an excellent description of each kind, at perhaps one-third of the cost charged even for inferior manufacture : a lady will thus be enabled not only to produce her own perfumes, (an elegant amusement, if a small still be used,) but she will obtain an abundant supply at a small expense, which, when the income is limited, must be an object worthy of attention.

All ladies are aware of the value of honey-water in cleansing the hair : we have given two recipes which will produce it in a far superior state to that commonly sold.

Having well cleansed the hair, the *Palma Christi*, No. 11, used according to the directions, will tend much to thicken and strengthen it. All are, we believe, aware of the superior properties of the Macassar Oil, or, if not, Mr. Rowland's advertisements will inform them. We have given a recipe (No. 12, Appendix) for producing it. We are informed, it is a genuine one, but cannot vouch for it: it is a nourishing, and yet stimulating oil, which is likely to be useful. Bear's-grease, No. 13, and the recipe No. 14, are excellent applications to prevent baldness : each of the other receipts may be applied for the purpose for which they are intended.

If the hair does not require thickening or strengthening, the free use of the brush, the occasional use of the honey-water to cleanse the hair, and a liberal use of one of the oils or pomades, will keep the hair in the highest state of perfection. Some hair does not, however, require much assistance from oils and pomades ; then, of course, these will not be wanted in the same quantity. When these aids are wanting, they must be used freely and regularly to produce any good effect.

To the Appendix we must refer our readers for several other particulars respecting the hair : these accompany the recipes.

Depilatories are preparations for removing superfluous hair. The recipes Nos. 38 and 39 are of this character. In using, we must caution our fair readers not to apply them to the little tufts of hair which sometimes appear upon moles ; the medical property of these drugs is powerfully stimulant, and somewhat caustic : the recipe No. 49 is very powerful ;

and as it contains orpiment, we must request them to be cautious in applying it : the part only from which the hair is wished to be removed must be touched, and a very small quantity of the mixture is required.

DISEASES OF THE HAIR, or rather of the head, are too dangerous to be trifled with. The most common are ring-worm and scald head, for we cannot call baldness a disease.

RING-WORM and scald head may generally be traced to disarrangement of the digestive organs, unless they have been acquired by contagion : particular attention to the general health should, therefore, accompany all local applications. We need scarcely say that *cleanlines and care* are most imperatively demanded in these diseases. While we strongly advise medical aid, we are aware that they can be cured without it ; but we have seen most frightful cases arise out of the attempt. Unprofessional persons can never know; until it is too late, whether they are doing good or harm ; consequently their practice is literally upon the principle of kill or cure.

The recipe No. 50 is a good local application ; but having mercury in its composition, it is dangerous in the hands of the uninitiated. The same may be said of what is purchased at the shops under the name of Edinburgh Ointment ; it is useful, but, being powerful, it is dangerous when the persons using it do not know whether they are doing good or harm. Tar-water, and tobacco-water, have each their advocates ; and, indeed, no single wash or ointment does much good, after having oeen used eight or ten days, as the eruption becomes accustomed to its stimul us.We have known a severe case of scald-head cured simply by the following process. The preliminary care here mentioned must always be attended to, and, at the same time, attention to the general health is absolutely necessary.

First, then, the loose dry scales, or excrescences, must be carefully removed, and the head washed with soap and water. This operation must be performed morning and evening : one instance of neglect will destroy all the advantages of a week's attention. The hair, also, which can be removed without pain, should be gently drawn out. After this and the washing, the lotion No. 102 should be applied.

After adopting this lotion for a week, try that marked 50 ; then, if the disease has not abated, apply No. 102 again, or either of the waters before-mentioned ; observing, however, never to continue the use of a wash that disagrees with the head. Great attention may be necessary to discover this.

Although the above practice has been successful, it may fail ; indeed, this disorder will continue for months to baffle the highest talent; we, therefore, once more repeat, apply to your medical attendant, if such a disorder obtains entrance into your house. For a long experience has led us to the conclusion that the best customers of the medical men are those who have the notion that they can cure themselves : the practice of a life will not make even a medical man acquainted with every aspect of disease ; how, then, is it likely that the small experience of a private nursery can qualify any person to combat with such an obstinate disease as that under consideration? A man who may have studied pharmacy, and, in addition, become acquainted with the entire anatomical theory, is still unfit to administer drugs in general practice, as he has still to learn the aspects which indicate the approach to recovery, which show a demand for tonics, stimulants, and the various means of the Pharmacopœia. "A little learning is a dangerous thing," and more especially so when applied to medicine and disease.

4

CHAPTER XI.

" IT is not sufficient," says a modern writer, " for the skin to be actually beautiful ; it must likewise appear so." It is quite certain that a judicious choice of colors in dress may heighten its lustre, and that want of judgment may totally destroy the appearance of the finest complexion. The judicious choice of color is, then, essential for the exhibition of beauty in its most exalted state of perfection.

A color, be it recollected, may be very beautiful in itself, but still completely opposed to the complexion of the person who is to wear it; when this is the case, it is absurd indeed to have a dress or a shawl which would have so injurious an effect upon the appearance. We fear, however, that the demands of fashion would be even more imperative than those of the intrinsic beauty of a vestment. Our readers cannot have failed to remark that when a particular color is the fashion, how very general is its adoption. Dark or fair, with a full color or a pale face, all will have it, whether it renders them frights or goddesses ; it is the fashion—" better be out of the world than out of the fashion ;" have it, all will, let it be ever so much opposed to their carnation.

The unobservant can scarcely conceive the effect which may be produced, how much beauty may be heightened, plain features improved, by a judicious selection of colors. A robe or a shawl may make or mar a complexion (we mean, of course, only for the time it is worn). How strange, then, that this circumstance should be so much disregarded !

A few hints upon this subject may not, then, be amiss. Ladies of fair complexion may even wear the purest white ; they should, in the choice of colors, select such as are light and brilliant,—rose, blue, or, if there be a slight tinge of brown in the carnation, light yellow ; be it, however, observed, that a perfectly light complexion would become almost livid by being opposed to yellow. Bright colors brighten a light com plexion, dark ones would give it the appearance of alabaster, destroy its life, and leave it without expression ; on the contrary, if light colors were opposed to a dark complexion, it would appear dull, lifeless, and inanimate ; the most suitable color for this is some of the varieties of yellow. Amber, for instance, is peculiarly suitable ; violet, puce, dark blue, purple, dark green, or even black, make it appear more fair, become animated, and enable it frequently to bear away the palm from its blonde competitors.

We have thought it advisable to say a few words upon dress in this work, but it was not our intention to go into the question of gracefulness in the adaptation of the clothes, although it certainly comes within the scope of our title.

The fashion of the form of a dress is frequently followed without any regard to the propriety of its adoption ; but this is quite contrary to good taste. Nothing can look much more absurd than a short stout figure adorned with a superfluity of flounces and trimmings, yet the power of fashion forces such exhibitions into continual notice ; even when fashion has decreed the flounces and trimmings shall be worn, such a figure need not be made ridiculous, and be made to bear as near as possible a resemblance to the prince of a Christmas dinner-table ; in such a case let the trimmings be placed as low as possible, and the dress be made very long ; the body also should be as long as convenient, and be made to fit tight. If the dress then hangs in graceful folds, it will add much to the appearance of length.

The arrangements of the upper part of the person can also be made to add to, or to diminish the height. Much trimming about the neck of a short stout person must make her look shorter ; her object should be to elongate the appearance of the neck, and thus further destroy the appearance of a superfluity of substance. Nature is especially kind to the 'adies in giving them so many personal advantages. Their hair offers them another means of apparently increasing their stature ; in so doing care must be taken not to raise the head-dress disproportionately, as to the above figure it would give the appearance of a mountain stuck upon a pigmy ; it should, however, be elevated in some measure, and at the same time diminished as much in breadth as will be consistent with the features, for we must not destroy a charm while we are attempting to remedy an evil.

All parts, indeed, of a lady's dress may be made to improve her figure or her face ; nor is the bonnet the least important,—how many pretty faces have been spoiled by an ugly bonnet ! fashion being the only thing attended to ; a good taste will

enable a person to avoid this. The trimmings may be generally so arranged as to suit a face by making the fashion
meet them half way ; if fashion dictate an absurdly large or
small bonnet, which is inappropriate to a certain physiognomy
let such a person adopt that degree of addition or diminution
which will be sufficient to be within the bounds of fashion
without spoiling her appearance, and she may depend that the
" graceful " will always ensure more admirers than the fashionable.

Everything that we have said upon a short figure must of
course be reversed with a tall one. Trimmings and flounces
may be adopted *ad libitum ;* the dress should be made full,
and the lines being broken by the flounces, the height of the
figure will be diminished ; if this is required to be done still
more, the dress should not reach the ground ; thus the eye
stops as it were in its survey, and the artifice is not perceived.

Everything we have said must be evident to the most ordinary observer ; but there are some persons who pass through
the world without observation ; there are others that have
little opportunity for observation, to these we address ourselves in these cursory remarks. The woman of the world is
aware that not only height and complexion and countenance
are affected by dress, but that it is capable of giving character
to the most insipid, of giving an air of command to natural in-
significance ; hence she dresses for the object she may have
in view ; every article of her apparel harmonizes, or is so opposed to another, as to produce an effect,—habit and tact are
generally sufficient for this. In our *little tome,* before mentioned, we have endeavored to assist this tact by illustrating
the principles by which these effects are produced ; so that a
lady may know why she looks well in this or the other—why
a certain dress is beautiful by natural light, and dull by an artificial light ; hundreds and thousands who are aware of such
facts have not the least idea of their cause ; hence they gain
little knowledge which can be available in circumstances dif-
fering from those in which they have heretofore been placed.
We hope to be a means of remedying this evil.

CHAPTER XII.

WE have already expressed our opinion respecting paints and cosmetics: the latter cannot, of course, be objected to when the name is only expressive of their quality ; but very many compositions which have this alluring title, prove after a while to be destroyers rather than beautifiers. When no improper substance is in a cosmetic, to use it or not is a mere matter of taste : the recipes we have given are all of this character ; and we can recommend them when their, or other assistance is determined upon. We confess to an old-fashioned admiration of natural and unassisted beauty.

Paints, however, can be of no benefit further than to produce a false appearance of beauty, and to a certain extent they must be injurious ; if even no poisonous ingredient be in their composition, because they fill up the pores of the skin, and if they do not prevent, they retard transpiration. But some of the fair sex may say, We cannot, or we will not submit to your training ; it is too late, or it is too tiresome ; can you not advise us of such paints as will be the least injurious ? Supposing ourselves thus addressed, we will, as in duty bound, obey, premising that if ablutions and friction are necessary to those who attend to our general system, (to those, therefore, who require not the assistance of paints,) they are imperatively demanded by those who do not. If our fair readers will attend to this, and use only such as we direct, we will insure them from any serious injury to health. We, must, however, warn them against using any metallic colors ; those which have white or red lead for their base, may, and often do, produce paralysis ; and many an ancient lady has received a paralytic stroke through this unsuspected cause. Sir Astley Cooper mentions the case of an eminent artist who applied to him to be treated for paralysis, and upon inquiry he found that he was in the habit of using a preparation of lead in some of his colors, and frequently rubbed it in with his finger ; by leaving off this habit the artist recovered. This case will serve to show the dangerous character of such preparations. To the Appendix we refer our readers for such colors as are the most innocent: each color is accompanied by remarks or explanations.

GENERAL REMARKS.

We shall now close our little volume by a few general remarks. The most superficial will at once acknowledge, that without health beauty cannot last, but must soon be impaired. The celestial beauty we have seen in consumptive persons, impresses us, even while we gaze, with the certainty of its evanescent nature ; that, too beautiful for earth, it will soon be transported to the immediate presence of the God that gave it. This beauty does not then militate against our hypothesis ; how strange then is it that, though all are convinced of the fact, so few will take the trouble to secure that reservoir of beauty which it is in the power of most to acquire.

We hope for success, as we have addressed ourselves to the feelings of mothers, and have shown them how they may secure to their offspring the greatest amount of physical beauty of which it is susceptible ; nay, more, as the mental powers are more active in health, the probability is that the attention to the physical may secure a superior intellectual development.

We hear a great deal of nonsense about the talented being sickly, and that the high intellect wears out its corporeal abode; such cases are and have been, but only exist where the principle of life has been originally weak ; the ardent spirit may then indeed destroy its sickly companion, but this is no more than is natural ; we see it throughout the world—the strong triumphing over the weak. But let the physical powers be cultivated, the mind participates in their health ; and the parent who judiciously attends to the health of her child, may reasonably hope that its intellect will become strong as its physical powers increase ; we, of course, are supposing that the child has the usual amount of talent.

Our remarks are, however, directed not merely to mothers as such, but to ladies in general—to them we say, that the importance of the fact warrants us again in drawing their attention to the system of ablution and friction we have recommended. To adopt it in part is all but useless ; the whole surface of the person must be passed over at least once a-day with either cold or tepid water. In the morning it refreshes and invigorates ; at night nature appears to rejoice in the act, as it almost invariably insures immediate and undisturbed sleep. In the winter it produces a glow, in the summer a delightful coolness ; it assists transpiration ; and while sleep has taken possession of the senses, it enables nature to perform effectually those mysterious processes by which she removes all impurities, and gives life and tone to the surface of the skin. It is also one of the greatest safeguards from colds. Water, as we have said, must be succeeded by friction ; this is more necessary in some constitutions than others. In cold weather it assists the return of warmth after a cold ablution ; it removes any excrescences which may have arisen on the surface, and by stimulating the skin, enables nature to completely clear its pores. The comfort derived from the act is unspeakable—it is a luxury to which, when once accustomed, you return at each stated period with the same desire and expectation as to the more ordinary sources of recruiting the exhausted powers ; the meals will, in time, not be more desired or expected than these ablutions and frictions. Beauty, comfort, and cleanliness are thus united. Here, then, is a source of delight, of which each lady may be possessed ; being convinced of the truth of our theory, and of the excellency of the practice, having observed its operation upon the health and appearance of those who have adopted it, we with confidence recommend it to our fair readers.

We had concluded, but the printer demands a few more lines to make the chapter fill out the page, and we are compelled at once to furnish them, without time to observe what elements of beauty we have left unnoticed—the temper and the various features we have already spoken of. It occurs to us that troublesome coughs, which drive away sleep at night, are sad enemies to beauty. We refer to a bronchial cough, commonly known as a throat cough, and we will therefore give a recipe for its removal, if early taken ; the stomach must however be attended to.

Take pil. styraci conp. 1½ drachm.

Pulv. ipecac. grs. xviii. ;

Divide into 24 pills, and take one, night and morning.

APPENDIX.

CONTAINING RECIPES FOR IMPROVING THE COMPLEXION—THE HAIR—THE HANDS—THE FEET—THE EYES—AND THE TEETH,—WITH A COLLECTION OF USEFUL MISCELLANIES.

DISTILLING.

GENERAL DIRECTIONS.

ALL perfumes should be distilled, which may be done by using a glass retort, with a napkin wetted with cold water covering the tube, attached to a receiver, placed upon a table, having an argand lamp burning under the retort, at a moderate distance, taking care that the liquid never runs, but that it passes drop by drop; when you perceive it inclined to run, remove the lamp to a greater distance. Very convenient stills for making perfumes, may be purchased at most mathematical instrument-makers; these perform the operation in a much more elegant manner than the above awkward contrivance; they are also more manageable and less liable to accident.

RECIPES FOR PERFUMES.

No. 1.—*Eau de Cologne.*

Take 38 drops of essence of cedral, 38 do. of bergamotte, 60 do. of oranges, 38 do. of citron 32 do. of neroli, 26 do. of Romain, 26 do. of meline, 1 pint of spirits of wine, 30 degrees above proof. Mix and distil.

No. 2.—*Eau de Cologne.*

Mix essence of bergamotte, lemon, lavender, and orange-flower water, of each 1 drachm; essence of cinnamon, ½ a drachm, spirits of rosemary, and honey-water, each two ounces; spirits of wine, 1 pint. Let the mixture stand a fortnight, then distil.

No. 3.—*Honey Water.*

Take 2½ ozs. of coriander seeds, ground small in a starch mill, a few slips of sweet marjoram in flower, dried and stripped from the twigs, 1 drachm of Calamus aromaticus, 1 drachm of yellow-saunders, and 1 drachm of orange and lemon peel ιet the three last-named articles be separately beaten to a fine powder.

Mix the above ingredients, and put them into a still that will hold three pints, and add to them 1 pint of rain water, 1 pint of proof spirit. Lute well all the joints of the apparatus, and leave the ingredients in this state without fire for 48 hours. At the end of this time, begin to distil by a very gentle heat, or the flowers and seeds will rise in the still head, stop up the worm, and spoil the process. Increase the fire after the first half-hour, and keep it at a regular heat till the termination of the process.

No. 4.—Honey Water.

Take 1 ounce of essence of bergamotte, 3 drachms of oil of lavender, ½ a drachm of oil of cloves, ½ a drachm of aromatic vinegar, 6 grains of musk or ambergris, 1½ pint of spirits of wine. Mix and distil according to above directions. Very superior perfume may be thus made. For removing superfluous hair, Nos. 48 and 49.

No. 5.—Odor delectabilis.

Take four ounces of distilled rose water, 4 do. of orange-flower water, 1 drachm of oil of cloves, 1 drachm of oil of lavender, 2 drachms of oil of bergamotte, 2 grains of ambergris, 2 grains of musk, and 1 pint of spirits of wine. Dissolve the musk and ambergris in the spirit of wine, then mix the whole well. It will be the better for being passed over a still.

No. 6.—Hungary Water.

To 1 pint of highly rectified spirits of wine, put an ounce of oil of rosemary, and 2 drachms of essence of ambergris : shake the bottle well several times, and let the cork remain out 24 hours. Cork the bottle, and then, after a month, during which time shake it daily, put the water into small bottles.

No. 7.—Lavender Water.

Take a pint of spirit of wine, essential oil of lavender, one ounce, essence of ambergris, two drachms ; put all into a quart bottle and shake extremely well.

No. 8.—Aromatic Vinegar.

Take 1 ounce of dried tops of rosemary, 1 ounce of dried leaves of sage, 1 ounce of dried flowers of lavender, 1 drachm of cloves, 1 drachm of camphor, 1½ pint of distilled vinegar Macerate for fourteen days, with heat, and then filter.

4*

No. 9.—*Aromatic Spirit of Vinegar.*

Take of the flowers of aromatic and perfumed shrubs, such as are directed for aromatic vinegar, No. 8, and digest them in strong vinegar, add a ¼ of a pint of spirits of wine to each pint of the infusion of vinegar, and then distil the composition.

No. 10.—*Lavender Water.*

Take 1 ounce of oil of lavender and bergamotte, 1 pint of rectified spirits of wine, 4 cloves bruised. Shake the above well, let it stand a month, then add 2 ounces of distilled water, and if you wish to retain its perfume, add 1 scruple of essence of musk, or ambergris, and distil the mixture.

RECIPES FOR IMPROVING THE HAIR.

No. 11.—*Palma-Christi Oil, for thickening the Hair.*

Take 1 ounce of Palma-Christi oil, add oil of lavender or bergamotte to scent it.

Let it be well brushed into the hair twice a day for two or three months, particularly applying it to those parts where it may be most desirable to render the hair luxuriant. This is a simple and valuable oil, and not in the hands of any monopolist.

No. 12.--*Macassar Oil.*

There is, in fact, no such thing imported into the country, although many thousands of pounds are annually expended, both in the advertising and in the purchasing of an article which passes under the name. The ingredients of which it is composed are the most simple and economical. The following, we are told, is the genuine recipe :—Take 1 quart of olive oil, 2½ ounces of spirits of wine, 1 ounce of cinnamon powder, 5 drachms of bergamotte. Heat them together in a large pipkin, then remove it from the fire, and add 4 small pieces of alkanet root; keep it closely covered for six hours, let it then be filtered through a funnel lined with blotting or filtering paper.

No. 13.—*An excellent Water to prevent Hair falling off, and to thicken it.*

Put 1 pound of unadulterated honey into a still, with 3 handsful of the tendrils of vine and the same quantity of rosemary tops. Distil as cool and as slowly as possible. The liquor may be allowed to drop till it tastes sour.

No. 14.—*Excellent Hair Oil to prevent Baldness*

Boil ½ a pound of green southernwood in 1½ pint of sweet

ofl, add ½ a pint of port wine. When boiled strain it through
a fine linen bag three times ; each time adding fresh southernwood, then add 2 ounces of bear's grease, and replace it near
the fire in a covered vessel, until the bear's grease be dissolved
Take it off, thoroughly mix the ingredients, and bottle it close.

No. 15.—To thicken the Hair.
Dip the tooth of your comb every morning in the expressed
juice of nettles, and comb the hair the wrong way. For the
same purpose some persons recommend the head to be shaved
and then fomented with a decoction of wormwood, southernwood, sage, betony, vervain, marjoram, myrtle, dill, rosemary
or mistletoe.

No. 16.—For darkening the Hair.
Wash the head with spring water, and comb the hair in the
sun, having dipped the comb in oil of tartar. Do this about
three times a day, and in less than a fortnight the hair usually
becomes quite black. The leaves of the wild vine, infused in
water, are also said to render the hair black, and to prevent its
falling off. Some persons use a metallic comb, which imparts
a dark shade to the hair ; they are now generally kept by the
perfumers, but it is a dirty habit.

No. 17.—To dye the Hair Flaxen.
We have heard the following is effective :
Take a quart of lye prepared from the ashes of vine twigs,
briony, celandine roots, and turmeric, of each ¼ an ounce, saf-
fron and lily roots, of each 2 drachms, flowers of mullein, yellow stechas, broom, and St. John's wort, of each a drachm.
Boil these together and strain off the liquor clear. Frequently
wash the hair with this fluid, and it will change it (we are told,)
in a short time, to a beautiful flaxen color.

No. 18.—Hair Dye.
We have seen the following recommended. We fear it
would injure the skin and turn it black if not used with great
care.
Take 2 drachms of silver, ¼ an ounce of steel filings ; pour
upon these 1 ounce of nitric acid, and let it remain until these
be dissolved, then add 8 ounces of rain water ; shake all well
together, and let it remain for 24 hours, then the floating liquor
will constitute the dye, and is to be applied with the hair-brush.

N. B. This is a caustic dye, and care must be taken that it
does not drop on the clothes.

No. 19.—Grecian Water for darkening the Hair

Dissolve two drachms of nitrate of silver in 6 ounces of distilled water, and add 2 drachms of gum water; perfume it to the taste, and wet the hair which is to be changed. If this touches the skin it will turn it black; though it does darken the hair at first, the black coloring will sometimes become purple. This mixture is generally sold at a very exhorbitant price.

RECIPES FOR IMPROVING THE COMPLEXION.
No. 20.—Cold Cream.

Take 2 drachms of white wax, 2 drachms of spermaceti, 2 ounces of hog's-lard; put altogether into a jar, which place into boiling water and stir till all is melted; take it out of the water and stir till nearly cold, then pour the mixture into rose water, and with the hand work it thoroughly, changing the water until the cream is very white. Return it to the jar, and as soon as it is melted, add 1 drachm of oil of almonds, and any perfume you approve. Let these be thoroughly incorporated, then remove it. When cold, put it up in rose water; if you wish to keep it in the greatest perfection, change the rose water every day.

No. 21.—Lady E. Conyngham's Face, or Lip Honey.

Take 2 ounces of fine honey, 1 ounce of purified wax, ¼ an ounce of silver litharge, and ¼ an ounce of myrrh. Mix over a slow fire, and add milk of roses, eau de Cologne, or any perfume you may prefer.

No. 22.—Almond Paste.

Take an ounce of bitter almonds, 1 ounce of barley flour, and honey a sufficient quantity to make the whole into a smooth paste.

No. 23.—Freckle Wash.

Take 1 drachm of muriatic acid, ¼ a pint of rain water, ¼ a tea-spoonful of spirit of lavender. Mix them well together, and apply two or three times a-day to the freckles, with a camel's-hair brush.

No. 24.—Purifying Water for the Skin.

Take 1 tea-spoonful of liquor of potassa, 2¼ ounces of pure water, a few drops of Eau de Cologne. Mix and apply as above.

No. 25.—Dr. Withering's Cosmetic Lotion.
Take a tea-cupful of cold sour milk ; scrape into it a quantity of horse radish. This must stand from six to twelve hours ; and then, being well strained, let it be applied, as directed on p. 44, two or three times a day.

No. 26.—Preventive Wash for Sunburn.
Take 2 drachms of borax, 1 drachm of Roman alum, 1 drachm of camphor, ¼ an ounce of sugar-candy, 1 pound of ox-gall. Mix and stir well together, and repeat the stirring three or four times a-day, until it becomes transparent. Then strain it through filtering or blotting paper, and it will be fit for use. Wash the face with the mixture before you go into the sun.

No. 27.—Grape Lotion for Sunburn.
Dip a bunch of green grapes in a basin of water ; sprinkle it with powdered alum and salt mixed ; wrap the grapes in paper, and bake them under hot ashes ; then express the juice, and wash the face with the liquid, which will usually remove either freckles, tan, or sunburn.

No. 28.—Lemon Cream for Sunburn and Freckles.
Put 2 spoonsful of sweet cream into ½ a pint of new milk ; squeeze into it the juice of a lemon, add half a glass of genuine French brandy, a little alum and loaf sugar ; boil the whole, skim it well, and when cool, it is fit for use.

No. 29.—Dr. Bateman's Sulphur Wash.
Break 1 ounce of sulphur, and pour over it one quart of boiling water ; allow it to infuse for twelve or fourteen hours, and apply it to the face two or three times a day, for a few weeks. This application is equally useful in removing that roughness of the skin which generally succeeds pimples. A more powerful application is sometimes prepared with vinegar and the acetated liquor of ammonia, or the spirit of mindere-rus. Or, the following, which will be equally effective, and known as—

No. 30.—Sir William Knighton's Lotion.
Half a drachm of liquor of potassa, 3 ounces of spirits of wine to be applied to the pimples with a camel's-hair brush, and if too powerful, add ¼ an ounce of cold water, which has been boiled and strained ; distilled water is better.

No. 31.—Pimple Ointment
Take 6 drachms of mercury, 6 grains of flour of sulphur, 2 ounces of hog's-lard ; mix carefully in a mortar.

N. B.   After applying any mercurial preparation, **be careful** not to get wet or exposed to drafts.

No. 32.—*Mr. Plumbe's Pimple Wash.*

Dissolve 2½ grains of oxymuriate of mercury in 4 ounces of spirits of wine : keep close in a phial with a glass stopper.

No. 33.—*Strawberry Lotion.*

Put into a pint bottle, ½ a pint of brandy, and as many strawberries as the brandy will cover, close the mouth of the bottle with a piece of bladder, and let it remain exposed to the sun for a week ; then strain it through a linen cloth, add as many more strawberries as the liquid will cover, and add ½ an ounce of camphor ; soak a pledget of lint in the mixture, and apply it to the parts.

No. 34.—*Liquor Plumbi.*

In the following proportions :—liquor plumbi 1 drachm, distilled water 1 ounce.
N. B.   This is an excellent lotion for allaying itching and inflammation.

No. 35.—*Court Plaster.*

Make a strong tincture of benzoin with spirits of wine, and add a weak solution of isinglass ; after making the silk moderately hot, strain it upon a roller and rub it over with this solution till it quite fills all the interstices of the silk ; when it has slowly dried, rub it with a solution of resin turpentine in tincture of benzoin, and let it remain stretched until perfectly dry.

No. 36.—*For Removing Wrinkles.*

Take 2 ounces of the juice of onions, 2 ounces of the white lily, 2 ounces of Narbonne honey, and 1 ounce of white wax ; put the whole into a new earthen pipkin until the wax is melted, then take the pipkin off the fire, and continue stirring briskly until it grows cold.   This should be applied on going to bed, and allowed to remain on till the morning.

No. 37.—*Lotion for Wrinkles.*

Take of the second water of barley 1 pint, and strain through a piece of fine linen, add a dozen drops of the balm of Mecca, shake it well together until the balm is thoroughly incorporated with the water, which will be effected when the water assumes a whitish or turgid appearance.   Before applying, wash the face with soft water ; we have heard, that if

used once a day it will beautify the face, preserve the freshness of youth, and give a surprising brilliancy to the skin. See
also Nos. 65, 66, 67, 68, 69, 78, and 79.

RECIPES FOR TOOTH POWDERS, &c.

No. 38.—*Aromatic Tooth Powder.*
Take finely powdered prepared chalk, 2 drachms, pure
starch, 2 drachms, myrrh, 2 drachms, ginger, ½ a drachm,
cuttle-fish bones, 2 drachms ; flower of lavender, and sugar at
pleasure, and mix well together.

No. 39.—*Camphor Paste.*
Take 1 ounce of boll ammoniac, 4 drachms of camphor ; let
the above be very finely powdered, then mix it with sufficient
honey to make it into a smooth paste, triturate it until entirely smooth. This is a most excellent paste for preserving and
beautifying the teeth. If a few drops of the tincture No. 41
be put into the water, and the tooth-brush dipped into it, it will
tend much to prevent tooth-ache.

No. 40.—*Tonic and Stimulating Dentifrice.*
Take 1½ drachm of powder of myrrh, 3 drachms of Peru-
vian bark, finely powdered, 10 drops of oil of cinnamon, 10
drops of oil of cloves, 1 ounce of prepared chalk, 2 drachms of
orris powder, 1 ounce of rose pink ; mix well together and
keep it close.

No. 41.—*Preservative Tincture for the Teeth and Gums.*
Take 4 drachms of camphor, 1 ounce of tincture of myrrh,
1 ounce of tincture of bark, and 1 ounce of rectified spirits of
wine ; mix them, and put 30 or 40 drops in a wine-glass of
water. Pour a little of this upon your brush before you apply
it to the powder, and when the teeth are clean, wash the
mouth, teeth and gums, with the remainder. It will in ordinary cases prevent tooth-ache.

No. 42.—*Powerfully Cleansing Dentifrice.*
Take fine powder of pumice-stone, 4 drachms, fine powder
of cuttle-fish bone, 4 drachms, ditto prepared chalk, 4 drachms ;
add one scruple of sub-carbonate of soda ; mix then well together, color and scent according to taste, and then pass it
through a fine sieve.

No. 43.—*Tonic and Anodyne Tooth Powder.*
Take fine powder of Florentine iris, 6 drachms, ditto pure
starch, 3 drachms, ditto quinine, 2 drachms, ditto hyoscyamus,

1 drachm; sugar to the taste, and perfume with otto of roses: carmine may be used to color it.

No. 44.—*Wash for the Teeth and Gums.*

Take the juice of half a lemon, a spoonful of rough claret or port wine, 10 grains of sulphate of quinine, a few drops of Eau de Cologne or oil of bergamotte; mix and keep in a well-stopped phial for use. For tooth-ache, see Nos. 87, 88 89, 90.

RECIPES FOR COLLYRIA OR EYE WATERS,
AND TO REMOVE INFLAMMATION FROM THE EYE-LID.

No. 45.—*Citrine Ointment.*

Take citrine ointment, 1 drachm, fresh lard, 3 drachms. Rub this on the eye-lids when going to bed, if the eye is inflamed from sitting up late.

No. 46.—*Anodyne Eye Water.*

Put 40 drops of the sedative solution of opium into 4 ounces of elder-flower water, and add 3 drachms of the best acetated liquor of ammonia; mix and apply it to the eye by means of a piece of fine linen, allowing some of the liquid to get under the eye-lid.

No. 47.—*Stimulating Eye Waters.*

Brandy, 2 drachms, water, 1 ounce. If it be not sufficiently strong, add a little more brandy; if, upon getting under the eye-lid, a slight pain is caused, it is strong enough; if acute pain, it is too strong.

Or, Take 3 grains of the acetate of zinc, 2½ ounces of rose-water, 3½ ounces of distilled water: mix.

RECIPES FOR DEPILATORIES;
OR TO REMOVE SUPERFLUOUS HAIR.

No. 48.—*Depilatory Vegetable Essence.*

Take polypody of the oak, cut into very small pieces, and put a quantity of it into a glass vessel; pour on this as much Lisbon or French white wine as will rise an inch above the ingredient, and place the vessel in hot water for 24 hours; then distil off the liquor, according to directions before given, but using hot water instead of the argand lamp; this water must of course be kept hot by placing a lamp under the vessel which contains it. Apply with a linen cloth, (which is to be kept on during the night) to the part from whence the hairs are to be removed. The oil of walnuts and the distilled waters of the leaves and roots of celandine are also said to bo efficacious.

No. 49.—*Depilatory Liniment.*

A more powerful Depilatory is thus made :—Take ¼ of a pound of gum ivy, dissolved in vinegar, 1 drachm of orpiment, and 2 drachms of gum Arabic, dissolved in the juice of hyoseyamus, in which ½ an ounce of quick lime has been dissolved. Make the whole into a liniment with a sufficient quantity of goose-grease, and apply a little to the part where you wish to destroy the hair. Be cautious in applying this.

No. 50.—*Camomile Lotion.*

Take ¼ a pint of strong chamomile tea, 15 drops of the liquor of oxymuriate of quicksilver ; mix and apply three times a day, particularly to old sores.

The water obtained at the coal-gas works is sometimes used successfully.

RECIPES FOR CHAPPED LIPS.
No. 51.—*Balsam for Chapped Lips.*

Take 2 spoonsful of clarified honey, with a few drops of lavender water, or any other more agreeable perfume. Mix, and anoint the lips frequently.

No. 52.—*For Chapped Lips.*

Put a ¼ of an ounce each of benjamin, storax, and spermaceti, two-pennyworth of alkanet-root, a large juicy apple chopped, a bunch of black grapes bruised, a ¼ of a pound of fresh butter, and 2 ounces of Bees-wax, into a new tin saucepan. Simmer gently till the wax, &c., are dissolved, and then strain it through a linen cloth. When cold, melt it again, and pour it into small pots or boxes. See also No. 21.

RECIPES FOR IMPROVING THE BREATH.
No. 53.—*Remedy for Bad Breath.*

Take 5 to 10 drops of hydrochloric acid in half a tumbler of spring water, a little lemon juice, and loaf sugar rubbed on lemon peel to flavor it to suit the palate. Let this mixture be taken three times a day for a month or six weeks, and if useful, then continued occasionally. It is a pleasant refrigerant and tonic draught.

No. 54.

When the breath is affected by constipation of the bowels, the following mixture will be useful :—

Take 4 drachms of Epsom salts, 8 drachms of tincture of Columba, 6 ounces of infusion of roses. Well shake the phial each time you take the draught, which should be every other morning, for a month or six weeks, a wine-glass full at each time.

No. 55.—Aperient and Tonic Draught for Fœtid Breath.

Take Epsom salts, 6 drachms, rhubarb in powder, 2 drachms, tincture of gentian, 1 ounce, compound infusion of roses, 3 ounces, distilled water, 4 ounces. Mix. Take 2 table-spoonsful, every morning or every other morning, an hour before breakfast for a month. See also Recipes from No. 91.

RECIPES FOR IMPROVING THE HANDS, FEET AND FOR REMOVING CORNS, WARTS, CHILBLAINS, AND CHAPS.

No. 56.—For Removing Warts.

Take of oxymuriate of mercury, 2 grains to 10, according to the strength you wish for ; lime water, 1 ounce. Mix and apply two or three times a day or oftener with a camel's-hair brush.

No. 56.—Solution of Nitrate of Silver.*

Take nitrate of silver, 1 drachm, pure water, 1 ounce. Apply to the warts very often with a camel's-hair brush.

No. 57.

Tinctura ferri sesquichloridi, 1 drachm. Apply to the warts with a camel's-hair pencil after having guarded the surrounding parts with court-plaster as directed to do when the nitrate of silver is applied, p. 56.

No. 58.—Soap for Chapped Hands.

Take 3 ounces of palm oil, 1 ounce of mutton suet, ½ of an ounce of white curd soap ; render down the suet, and work it well till it is as smooth as pomatum, then shave the soap fine and melt with the suet in a pipkin. When it is thoroughly melted, add the palm oil ; stir while it is simmering, and take it off the fire as soon as it is thoroughly mixed with the other ingredients. Pour the whole into a vessel and keep stirring till it is cool, or the soap will separate. Perfume to your taste. Rub this well into the hands on going to bed, (after having well washed and dried them,) then put a pair of white kid gloves, and it will very shortly make them soft, and entirely prevent chapping. Applied to the feet in the same way substituting a piece of linen instead of gloves, it prevents chilblains.

No. 59.—Chilblain Lotion.

Take liquor plumbi acetatis, 1 ounce, ½ a pint of cold water, add 1 glass of good brandy or rum. Mix, until it becomes of a uniform white. Apply the lotion with linen several times a day.

No. 59.*—Sir Astley Cooper's Chilblain Liniment.

Take liquor of subacetate of lead, 1 ounce, camphorated spirits of wine, 2 ounces ; mix, and rub into the hands or feet two or three times a day ; oftener if convenient.

N. B.—This is an excellent application, and well worthy of attention. Occasionally soak the feet in warm water going to bed, and then apply the liniment.

No. 60.—Acetate of Ivy.

Take ivy leaves fresh gathered, 1 ounce ; place them in a covered pomade pot or wide-mouthed bottle, which has a stopper. Cover them with vinegar ; and in a fortnight they will be fit to use ; add vinegar as it is absorbed. Place a part of the leaf upon the corn, and confine it there in any convenient manner. This is often very effective.

No. 61.—Infallible Corn Plaster.

Take 2 ounces of gum ammoniac, 2 ounces of yellow wax, 6 drachms of verdigris ; mix them together, and spread the composition on a piece of linen or soft leather, first rubbing down the corn with an instrument like a file ; it is to be purchased at most chemists. A file not too coarse will, however, answer the same purpose. Let the plaster be renewed in a fortnight, if necessary.

No. 62.—Mechanical Corn Plaster.

The best is bought at the shops : a substitute may be made by taking a piece of diachylon plaster somewhat larger than the corn ; cut a hole in the centre, sufficiently large to admit the corn through it ; warm the plaster and place it on the foot ; continue adding piece upon piece until the plaster is a shade higher than the top of the corn. The corn will thus be removed by the pressure of the shoe being taken from it.

No. 63.—Emollient Ointment for Chilblains.

Take Speer's opodeldoc, 2 oz., laudanum, 1 ounce ; mix. Anoint the parts night and morning. At night soak the feet

No. 64.—*To Prevent Chilblains.*
Make a strong solution of alum with cold water, and before
the winter comes on, repeatedly bathe the parts with this; to
render it more strengthening, you may add a small quantity of
infusion of galls or infusion of oak bark.

COMPLEXION—(*continued*).
No. 65.—*Bath of Modesty.*
Take 4 ounces of sweet almonds, peeled, 1 pound of pine-
apple kernels, 1 pound of elecampane, 10 handsful of linseed,
1 ounce of marsh mallow roots, 1 ounce of white lily roots.
Pound all these till reduced to a paste, and tie it up in several
small bags, which are to be thrown into a tepid bath, and
pressed till the water becomes milky.

No. 66.
A more simple method of preparing a bath of this kind, is
given by M. Moreau de la Sarthe, who says, it is sufficient
to throw into the bath a sufficient quantity of almonds made
into a paste, to give the water a milky appearance. Or, see
almond paste, Nos. 83, 84.

No. 67.—*Milk of Houseleek.*
Beat a quantity of houseleek in a marble mortar, squeeze
out the juice and clarify it. When you want to use it, pour a
few drops of rectified spirit on the juice, and it will instantly
turn milky. It is a very efficacious remedy for a pimpled
face, and preserves the skin soft and smooth.

No. 68.—*Virgin Milk.*
Take equal parts of gum benzoin and styrax, dissolve in a
sufficient quantity of spirits of wine, the spirits will then
become a reddish tincture, and exhale a very fragrant smell.
Some people add a little balm of Gilead. Drop a few drops
into a glass of clear water, and by stirring the water, it instantly changes milky. Ladies use it successfully to clear the
complexion.

No. 69.—*Cosmetic Juice.*
Make a hole in a lemon, fiill it with sugar-candy, and close
it with leaf gold, applied over the rind that was cut out; then
roast the lemon in hot ashes. When desirous of using the
juice, squeeze out a little through the hole already made, and
with it wash the face with a napkin. This juice is said to
cleanse the skin and brighten the complexion wonderfully

No. 70—*Soft Pomatum.*

Soak ½ a pound of unsalted fresh lard, and ¼ of a pound of beef marrow, in water two or three days, changing and beating it every day; put it into a sieve, and when drained, into a jar which place in a saucepan of water. Put the saucepan on a slow fire, and when the composition is melted, pour it into a basin and beat it with two spoonsful of brandy, drain off the brandy, and add essence of lemon, otto of roses, millefleur, or any scent you prefer.

RECIPES FOR PAINTS,
WHICH MAY BE USED WITHOUT DANGER.
No. 71.—*Carmine.*

Carmine is the finest red color we have. It comes chiefly from Germany; is made from cochineal, and is consequently simple. There are two or three sorts of this article. The finest, which bears a high price, is in the end by far the cheapest. The difference between the two sorts will not easily be discerned by mere inspection; besides, the intensity of the color renders it painful for the eye to dwell on, even for a minute. Comparison will point out a difference, but the surest way of detecting adulteration is to fill a silver thimble with each sort: the finest and best will not weigh above one-half or two-thirds of the worst, which is commonly mixed with vermilion or red lead, both of which are very heavy powders.

No. 72.—*Portuguese Rouge.*

Of Portuguese dishes, there are two sorts; one of these is made in Portugal, and is rather scarce; the paint contained in the dishes being of a fine pale pink hue, and very beautiful in its application to the face. The other is made in London, and is of a dirty red color; it may suit those who never saw the genuine Portuguese dishes. The most marked difference between the two sorts is, that the true one from Portugal is contained in dishes which are rough on the outsides, whereas those made here are glazed and quite smooth.

No. 73.—*Spanish Wool.*

Of this, there are several sorts, but that which is made in London is considered best; that which comes from Spain being of a very dark red, whereas the former is of a bright pale red, and when good, the cakes, which are usually the size of a half-crown, shine and glisten, between a green and gold color. This wool is best when made in hot, dry weather, for then it gives a brilliant color, but what is made in wet weather, is of a coarse dirty color. Besides the advantage of having it better, it can also be bought cheaper in summer, as in winter **the** maker is dependent on the weather.

No. 74.—*Spanish Papers.*

These papers are of two sorts; they differ from the above in nothing more than that in the former the color tinges the wool, and here it is laid on paper, chiefly for the convenience of carrying in a pocket-book. This colored wool comes from China, in large round cakes, about three inches in size. The finest of these impart a most agreeable tint to the cheek, but it is seldom possible to pick from a parcel more than three or four of a really fine color; for as the cakes are loose, the sea voyage and exposure to air, even in opening them to show a friend, carry off the most delicate tint.

No. 75.—*Chinese Boxes of Colors.*

These boxes, which are beautifully painted and japanned, come from China. They contain each two dozen papers, and in each paper are three smaller ones; viz., a small black paper for the eye-brows; another of a fine green color, but which, when fresh, makes a fine red for the face; and, a paper containing about half-an-ounce of white powder, (prepared from real pearl) for some parts of the face and neck.

These colors are not common, therefore the best way is to commission some friend who may be going to China, to purchase them. The red powders are best applied by a fine camel's-hair brush; the colors in the dishes, wools, and green papers, are commonly laid on by the tip of the little finger, previously wetted; but as gum is used in their composition, they are apt to leave a shining appearance on the skin.

No. 76.—*White Pearl Powder.*

The best white is literally *pearl powder, i. e.*, made from pearls; and this is as safe, as its effects are natural and beautiful. A most dangerous compound of bismuth is, however, sold under this name, against the use of which we have cautioned our fair readers. (See Introduction.) The next best is—

No. 77.—*Talc White.*

Take a piece of Briancon chalk; choose it of a pearl grey color, and rasp it gently with a piece of dog-skin: after this, sift it through a sieve of very fine silk, and put this powder into a pint of good distilled vinegar, in which leave it for a fortnight; shake the bottle every day except the last, on which it must not be disturbed; pour off the vinegar so as to **leave the chalk** behind in the bottle, into which **pour clear**

water that has been distilled or filtered ; throw the whole into a clean pan, and stir the water well with a wooden spatula ; let the powder settle again to the bottom, then pour the water gently off, and wash the powder six or seven times, taking care always to use filtered or distilled water. When the powder is as soft and white as you wish, dry it in a place where it is not exposed to the dust ; sift it through a silken sieve which will make it still finer. It may be either left in powder, or wetted and formed into cakes, like those sold by the perfumers. One pint of vinegar is sufficient to dissolve a pound of talc. This white is used by dipping the finger, or a piece of paper, or a hare's foot prepared for the purpose, in cold cream, and putting upon it about a grain of this white. which will not be removed even by perspiration.

<hr>

COMPLEXION—(continued).
No. 78.—Milk of Roses.

Take ½ a pound of Jordan almonds, 2½ pints of rose-water, ¼ of a pint of rectified spirits of wine, 1 drachm of oil of lavender, ¼ an ounce of Castile soap, and 1 ounce of cream of roses. Blanch the almonds in boiling water. dry them well in a cloth, and then pound them in a mortar till they become a complete paste. Pound the soap in the same mortar, and let it be well mixed with the almond paste. When this is done, add the cream of roses, mix again, and then with a spatula stir in the rose-water and spirits. Strain the whole through a clean white cloth, and add the oil of lavender to the expressed liquid, *drop by drop*, stirring it the whole time. When the mixture has stood a day, covered with a cloth to keep it from dust, it must be bottled.

No. 79.—Cold Cream.

Take 2 drachms of clear neat's-foot oil, 3 drachms of very white oil of jessamine, 1½ drachm of spermaceti, and one ounce of white wax scraped fine. Melt the whole gently, and mix very thoroughly, then pour it into a basin, which in winter must be kept warm by the fire. Then beat the whole with a wooden spoon without intermission till it becomes a consistent and very white body. Add 2 ounces of rose or orange-flower water, 6 drops of spirit of ambergris, bergamotte, or any other scent you prefer ; beat the mixture very thoroughly till the whole of the spirit and water is absorbed by the unctuous substances ; this will add greatly to the whiteness and richness of flavor of the cream, which, if care has been taken that all the utensils were perfectly clean and free from dust, will, in this stage of the process, be as white as snow.

N. B.—In making cold cream in winter, great care must be

taken that all the utensils for the preparation are kept warm, and the rose or orange-flower water warmed before added to the cream, or it will congeal and oblige the operator to melt the whole again. In summer, on the contrary, everything must be kept as cool as possible, and more wax used in proportion, according to the state of the weather. When put into pots, a few drops of honey-water on the top will greatly improve the flavor and keep it cool by evaporation.

No. 80.—*Pomade Divine, for Bruises, Rheumatism, &c.*

Take 1½ pounds of beef marrow; after clearing it from the strings and pieces of bone, place it in a vessel of spring water; let it remain ten days, changing it twice daily, steep it in rose water twenty-four hours, and then drain it in a cloth till quite dry. Take styrax, gum benjamin, odoriferous cypress-powder, of each 1 ounce, ½ an ounce of cinnamon, 2 drachms of cloves, and 2 drachms of nutmegs, all in fine powder; mix them with the marrow, and put them altogether into a pewter-pot that holds three pints; cover the top of the pot very close that the steam does not evaporate; place the pot into a large vessel of boiling water, but observe to keep it steady, and as the water shrinks add more quite boiling, for it must boil four hours without ceasing a minute. Strain the ointment through a fine linen cloth into small pots, and when cold cover them. Do not touch it with any metal but silver. It will keep many years.

RECIPES FOR SOAPS.

No. 81.—*Soap for Improving the Color.*

Dissolve 2 ounces of Venice soap in 2 ounces of lemon juice; add 1 ounce of oil of almonds, and 1 ounce of oil of tartar. Mix and stir it till it has acquired the consistence of honey.

No. 82.—*Musk Soap.*

Take 2 ounces of marsh mallow roots, cleaned and dried in the shade, reduce them to powder, add ½ an ounce of starch, do. of flour, 3 drachms of fresh pine-apple kernels, 1 ounce of orange pippins, 1 ounce of oil of tartar, and of oil of almonds, and a ½ of a drachm of musk. Reduce the dry ingredients to a very fine powder, and to each ounce of powder add ½ an ounce of Florence iris. Then steep 4 ounces of fresh roots, in orange-flower water, let them stand a night, squeeze them well, and with the mucilage that comes from them, make a paste with the powder. Let this paste dry and mould it into round balls. Nothing makes the hands softer or whiter.

No. 83.—Almond Paste for the Hands.

Take 1 pound of sweet almonds, a ¼ of a pound of bread crumbs. ¼ a pint of spring water, ½ a pint of brandy, and the yolks of two eggs. Pound the almonds with a few drops of vinegar or water, to prevent them oiling, add the crumbs of bread, which moisten with the brandy as you mix it with the almonds and the yolks of eggs. Set this mixture over a slow fire, and stir it continually, or it will adhere to the vessel.

No. 84.—Almond Paste for Chapped Hands, and which will preserve them smooth by constant Use.

Mix a quarter of a pound of unsalted hogs'-lard, which has been washed in common, and then in rose-water, with the yolks of two new-laid eggs, and a large spoonful of honey Add as much paste from almonds (well pounded in a mortar) as will work it into a paste.

No. 85.—Seraglio Soap.

Take ½ a pound of iris, 2 ounces of benzoin, ½ an ounce of storax, 1 ounce of yellow sanders, ½ a drachm of cinnamon, a few cloves, a little lemon peel, St. Lucia wood, and nutmeg. Well pulverize the whole: take about ½ a pound of white soap, grate it and put it to soak for four or five days, in a pint and a half of brandy, with the powder; knead up the whole with a quart of orange-flower water, make a paste of this soap, with a sufficient quantity of starch, form it into any shape you please, adding whites of eggs, and gum dragon, dissolved in any kind of scent you prefer.

No. 86.—To make Wash Balls.

Shave thin 2 pounds of new white soap into about a teacupful of rose water, then pour as much boiling water on as will soften it. Put into a brass pan a pint of sweet oil, fourpenny worth of oil of almonds, ½ pound of spermaceti, and set all over the fire till dissolved; then add the soap, and stir it till it begins to thicken slightly; then add essence of millefleurs, into which have been put 2 or 3 drops of ambergris (to make it retain its perfume). Continue stirring the whole till it is thick enough to roll up into hard balls, which must then be done as quickly as possible.

RECIPES TO REMOVE TOOTH-ACHE.

No. 87.—Lotion for Tooth-ache.

Put 2 drachms of camphor into an ounce of the oil of turpentine, and let it dissolve, when it will be fit for use.

No. 88.—Mucilage for the Tooth-ache.

Take 1 drachm of the powdered leaves of pyrethrum, and a sufficient quantity of gum arabic mucilage. Make a mass, divide it into twelve portions, and take one into the mouth, and let it lie till dissolved as occasion requires.

No. 88.*—Dr. Blake's Infallible cure for the Tooth-ache.

Take alum, reduced to an impalpable powder, 2 drachms; nitreous spirits of ether, 7 drachms. Mix and apply them to the tooth.

This is said to be an infallible cure for all kinds of Tooth-ache (unless the disease is connected with rheumatism).

No. 89.—Liniment for Tooth-ache.

Take an ounce of spirit of camphor, 3 drachms of liquor ammonia, 10 drops of essential oil of bergamotte. Mix them in a phial for use.

No. 89.*—Essence to remove the Tooth-ache.

Take 1 drachm of camphor, rectified spirits of wine, 2 drachms, opium, 5 grains, oil of box, or oil of cloves, 10 drops, gum guaiacum, 10 grains. Mix them, 4 or 5 drops, on lint, put into the hollow tooth, or if a sound one, 6 or 7 drops in the ear on the same side as the tooth affected, will remove the tooth-ache, unless it arises from the stomach being out of order, or from rheumatism, then the medicine must be taken; if not relieved, repeat it in half an hour.

N. B. All these may sometimes fail, if used too often; when either appears to have no effect, try one of the others.

No. 90.—Fomentation for the Face, to assist in relieving Tooth-ache.

Take three poppy-heads, a handful of chamomile flowers, put them into a quart of soft water; boil until the quart is reduced to about a pint, then apply it repeatedly to the face by means of flannel, and as hot as it can be borne. Take care no draught of air gets to the face while under its operation. For Tooth Powders, see No. 38 and following.

LAVEMENTS AND USEFUL MEDICINES AND MISCELLANIES.

No. 91.—Aperient Lavements.

Take warm water, three parts of a pint, Rochelle salts, 1 ounce, castor oil, 2 ounces.

No. 92.—A stronger one.

Take warm gruel, three parts of a pint, Epsom salts, 2 ounces. castor oil, 2 ounces.

No. 93.—Another.

Take warm gruel, three parts of a pint, infusion of senna, 3 ounces, Epsom salts, 1 ounce.

N. B.   In all cases where salts are used, dissolve the salts with a little of the warm water or gruel before the oil is added. The heat of the mixture should be such as you can pleasantly bear upon the back of the hand.

No. 94.—Aperient Pills.

Take compound extract of colocynth, 2 drachms, extract of hyoscyamus, 1 scruple, calomel, 12 grains, oil of peppermint, 5 drops.   Divide into 15 pills; take one or two occasionally at bedtime.

No. 95.—Spirit of Mindererus.

This may be purchased at the shops, under the name of the acetated spirit of ammonia.   It may be made thus: Take sub-carbonate of ammonia, $\frac{1}{4}$ ounce, diluted acetic acid, half a pint; mix.   It is a useful and cooling diaphoretic, and promotes a gentle perspiration.   Very useful in fevers.

No. 96.—Castor Oil.

From $\frac{1}{2}$ an ounce to an ounce is generally sufficient.   A convenient mode of taking it is thus: half-fill a wine-glass with weak brandy and water, then rub a little *brandy* upon the inside of the glass which is not occupied by the above; immediately after so doing, pour the oil gently upon the top of the brandy and water, and take it off quickly; by this means it will scarcely be tasted.   Some prefer taking it in coffee.   An excellent preparation is now sold by most chemists; it consists of castor oil enclosed in small capsules; these can be swallowed as pills, and of course are perfectly tasteless.

No. 97.—Stimulant, Aperient, and Tonic Draught.

Take carbonate of ammonia, 2 scruples, carbonate of soda, 2 drachms, compound infusion of senna, 3 ounces, infusion of Columba, 4 ounces, distilled water, 2 ounces.   Take two table-spoonfuls three times.

No. 98.—Aperient Mixture.

Take compound infusion of senna, $1\frac{1}{2}$ ounce, cinnamon water, 2 drachms, manna, 1 drachm, extract of liquorice, $\frac{1}{2}$ a scruple; mix.   The above is a mild, but effectual aperient.

No. 99.—*Tonic, Antacid, and mildly Aperient.*

Take sesquicarbonate of soda, 2 drachms, compound infusion of genetian, 4 ounces, compound infusion of senna, 4 ounces, mint water, 2 ounces.   Take two table-spoonfuls three times a day.

No. 100.—*Aperient Pills.*

Take Socotrine aloes, 1 drachm, Castile soap, 1 drachm, conserve of hips enough to form the mass, which divide into forty pills.   Take two once or twice a day.

No. 101.—*Tonic Pills.*

Take extract of gentian, 1 drachm, sulphate of quinine, 1 drachm; mix and divide into twenty-four pills.   Take one about two hours before dinner.

No. 102.—*Wash for Scald Head.*

Take ½ an ounce of sulphate of potass, 1 pint of lime water, 1 ounce of soap liniment; mix and apply to the head two or three times a day.

INDEX.

The Reason Why : General Science.

A careful collection of some thousands of reasons for things, which, though generally known, are imperfectly understood. A book of condensed scientific knowledge for the million. By the author of "Inquire Within." It is a handsome 12mo volume, of 356 pages, bound in cloth, gilt, and embellished with a large number of wood cuts, illustrating the various subjects treated of. This work assigns reasons for the thousands of things that daily fall under the eye of the intelligent observer, and of which he seeks a simple and clear explanation.

EXAMPLE.

Why does silver tarnish when exposed to the light? Why is the sky blue?
his volume answers 1,325 similar questions. Price................$1 50

The Biblical Reason Why.

A Hand-Book for Biblical Students, and a Guide to Family Scripture Readings. By the author of "Inquire Within," &c. Illustrated, large 12mo, cloth, gilt side and back. This work gives reasons, founded upon the Bible, and assigned by the most eminent Divines and Christian Philosophers, for the great and all absorbing events recorded in the History of the Bible, the Life of our Saviour, and the Acts of His Apostles.

EXAMPLE.

Why did the first patriarchs attain such extreme longevity?
Why is the Book of the Prophesies of Isaiah a strong proof of the authenticity of the whole Bible?
This volume answers upwards of 1,400 similar questions. Price....$1 50

The Reason Why : Natural History.

By the author of "Inquire Within," "The Reason Why," &c. 12mo, cloth, gilt side and back. Giving reasons for hundreds of interesting facts in connection with Zoology, and throwing a light upon the peculiar habits and instincts of the various Orders of the Animal Kingdom.

EXAMPLE.

Why do dogs turn around two or three times before they lie down?
Why do birds often roost upon one leg?
his volume answers about 1,500 similar questions. Price...........$1 50

The Sociable; or, One Thousand and One Home Amusements.

Containing Acting Proverbs, Dramatic Charades, Acting Charades, Tableaux Vivants, Parlor Games and Parlor Magic, and a choice collection of Puzzles, &c., illustrated with nearly 300 Engravings and Diagrams, the whole being a fund of never-ending entertainment. By the author of the "Magician's Own Book." Nearly 400 pages, 12mo, cloth, gilt side stamp. Price--$1 50

Inquire Within for Anything You Want to Know; or Over

3,700 Facts for the People. Illustrated. 436 large pages. Price.....$1 50

"Inquire Within" is one of the most valuable and extraordinary volumes ever presented to the American public, and embodies nearly 4,000 facts, in most of which any person will find instruction, aid and entertainment. It contains so many valuable recipes, that an enumeration of them requires seventy-two columns of fine type for the index.

The Corner Cupboard ; or, Facts for Everybody.

By the Author of "Inquire Within." Large 12mo, 400 pages, cloth, gilt side and back. Illustrated with over 1,000 Engravings. Price...........$1 50

Send cash orders to Dick & Fitzgerald, New York.

Chesterfield's Art of Letter-Writing Simplified.
A Guide to Friendly, Affectionate, Polite, and Business Correspondence. Containing a large collection of the most valuable information relative to the Art of Letter-Writing, with clear and complete instructions how to begin and end Correspondence, Rules for Punctuation and Spelling, &c., together with numerous examples of Letters and Notes on every subject of Epistolary Intercourse, with several important hints on Love-Letters. Price...12 cts.

Knowlson's Farrier, *and Complete Horse Doctor.* We have
printed a new and revised edition of this celebrated book, which contains Knowlson's famous Recipe for the Cure of Spavin, and other new matter. It is positively the best book of the kind ever written. We sell it cheap, because of the immense demand for it. The farmers and horse keepers like it because it gives them plain, common-sense directions how to manage their horses. We sell our new edition (64 pages, 18mo) cheap. Price...12 cts.

The Art of Conversation. With Remarks on Fashion
and Address. By Mrs. MABERLY. This is the best book on the subject ever published. It contains nothing that is verbose or difficult to understand, but all the instructions and rules for conversation are given in a plain and common-sense manner, so that any one, however dull, can easily comprehend them. 64 pages octavo, large. Price.......................25 cts.

Horse-Taming by a New Method, *as Practiced by*
J. S. Rarey. A New and Improved Edition, containing Mr. Rarey's whole Secret of Subduing and Breaking Vicious Horses, together with his improved Plan of Managing Young Colts, and Breaking them to the Saddle, the Harness and the Sulkey, with ten Engravings illustrating the process. Every person who keeps a horse should buy this book. It costs but a trifle, and you will positively find it an excellent guide in the management of that noble animal. This is a very handsome book of 64 pages. Price..12 cts.

The Game of Whist. Rules, Directions and Maxims to
be observed in playing it. Containing, also, Primary Rules for Beginners, Explanations and Directions for Old Players, and the Laws of the Game. Compiled from Hoyle and Matthews. Also, Loo, Euchre, and Poker, as now generally played. With an explanation of Marked Cards, &c., &c. Price...12 cts.

The Ladies' Love Oracle; *or, Counselor to the Fair Sex.*
Being a Complete Fortune Teller and Interpreter to all questions upon the different events and situations of life, but more especially relating to all circumstances connected with Love, Courtship and Marriage. By MADAMI LE MARCHAND. Beautifully illustrated cover, printed in colors. Price...30 cts

The Laws of Love. A Complete Code of Gallantry
Containing concise rules for the conduct of Courtship through its entire progress, aphorisms of love, rules for telling the characters and disposition of women, remedies for love, and an Epistolary Code. 12mo, paper. Price...25 cts

The Great Wizard of the North's Hand-Book o
Natural Magic. Being a series of the Newest Tricks of Deception, arranged for Amateurs and Lovers of the Art. By Professor J. H. ANDERSON the great Wizard of the North. Price.........................25 cts

Dr. Valentine's Comic Lectures; or, *Morsels of*
Mirth for the Melancholy. A budget of Wit and Humor, and a certain cure for the blues and all other serious complaints. Comprising Comic Lectures on Heads, Faces, Noses, Mouths, Animal Magnetism, Etc., with Specimens of Eloquence, Transactions of Learned Societies, Delineations of Eccentric Characters, Comic Songs, Etc., Etc. By Dr. W. VALENTINE, the favorite Delineator of Eccentric Characters. Illustrated with twelve portraits of Dr. Valentine, in his most celebrated characters. 12mo, cloth, gilt. Price..$1 25
Ornamental paper cover. Price..75 cts.

Dr. Valentine's Comic Metamorphoses. Being the
second series of Dr. Valentine's Lectures, with Characters, as given by the late Yankee Hill. Embellished with numerous portraits. Ornamental paper cover. Price...75 cts.
Cloth, gilt. Price..$1 25

Mrs. Partington's Carpet-Bag of Fun. A Collec-
tion of over one thousand of the most Comical Stories, Amusing Adventures, Side-Splitting Jokes, Cheek-Extending Poetry, Funny Conundrums, QUEER SAYINGS OF MRS. PARTINGTON, Heart-Rending Puns, Witty Repartees, Etc., Etc. The whole illustrated by about 150 comic wood cuts. 12mo, 300 pages, cloth, gilt. Price......................$1 25
Ornamented paper covers. Price......................................75 cts.

Sam Slick in Search of a Wife. 12mo, paper.
Price...75 cts.
Cloth. Price...$1 25
Everybody has heard of "Sam Slick, the Clockmaker," and he has given his opinion on almost everything.

Sam Slick's Nature and Human Nature. Large
12mo. Paper. Price...75 cts.
Cloth. Price...$1 25

The Attache; or, *Sam Slick in England.* 12mo. Paper.
Price...75 cts.
Cloth. Price...$1 25

Sam Slick's Sayings and Doings. Paper. Price 75 cts.
Cloth. Price...$1 25

Ladies' Guide to Crochet. By Mrs. ANN S. STEPHENS.
Copiously illustrated with original and very choice designs in Crochet, Etc., printed in colors, separate from the letter-press, on tinted paper. Also with numerous wood-cuts, printed with the letter-press, explanatory of terms, Etc. Bound in extra cloth, gilt. This is by far the best work on the subject of Crochet ever published. Price $1 25

The Laughable Adventures of Messrs. Brown,
Jones and Robinson. Showing where they went and how they went; what they did and how they did it. With nearly two hundred most thrillingly comic engravings. Price...30 cts.

The Knapsack Full of Fun; or, *One Thousand Rations*
of Laughter. Illustrated with over 500 comical Engravings, and containing over one thousand Jokes and Funny Stories. By DOESTICKS and other witty writers. Large quarto. Price...30 cts.

The Plate of Chowder; *A Dish for Funny Fellows.* Ap-
propriately illustrated with 100 Comic Engravings. By the author of "Mrs. Partington's Carpet-Bag of Fun." 12mo, paper cover. Price 25 cts.

The Bordeaux Wine and Liquor-Dealers' Guide.
A Treatise on the Manufacture of Liquors. By a Practical Liquor Manufacturer. 12mo, cloth. The author, after telling what each liquid is composed of, furnishes a formula for making its exact counterpart—exact in everything. Each formula is comprehensive—no one can misunderstand it. Price,--$2 50

The Ladies' Guide to Beauty. A Companion for the
Toilet. Containing practical advice on improving the complexion, the hair, the hands, the form, the teeth, the eyes, the feet, the features, so as to insure the highest degree of perfection of which they are susceptible. And also upwards of one hundred recipes for various cosmetics, oils, pomades, &c., &c. Paper. Price-- 25 cts.

Broad Grins of the Laughing Philosopher. Being
a Collection of Funny Jokes, Droll Incidents, and Ludicrous pictures. By PICKLE THE YOUNGER. This book is really a good one. It is full of the drollest incidents imaginable, interspersed with good jokes, quaint sayings, and funny pictures. Price--13 cts.

Yale College Scrapes ; or, How the Boys Go It at New
Haven. This is a book of 111 pages, containing accounts of all the noted and famous "Scrapes" and "Sprees," of which students at Old Yale have been guilty for the last quarter of a century. Price-------------25 cts.

The Comic English Grammar ; or, A Complete Grammar
of our Language, with Comic Examples. Illustrated with about fifty Engravings. Price--25 cts.

The Comical Adventures of David Dufficks.
Illustrated with over one hundred Funny Engravings. Large octavo. Price --25 cts.

BOUND SONG BOOKS.

Tony Pastor's Complete Budget of Comic Songs
Containing a complete collection of the New and Original Songs, Burlesque Orations, Stump Speeches, Comic Dialogues, Pathetic Ballads, as sung and given by the celebrated Comic Vocalist, TONY PASTOR. Cloth gilt. Price--$1 25

The Universal Book of Songs. Containing a choice
collection of 400 new Sentimental, Scotch, Irish, Ethiopian and Comic Songs. 12mo, cloth, gilt. Price----------------------------------$1 25

The Encyclopedia of Popular Songs. Being a com
pilation of all the new and Fashionable Patriotic, Sentimental, Ethiopian Humorous, Comic and Convivial Songs, the whole comprising over 40 songs. 12mo, cloth, gilt. Price----------------------------------$1 25

The Lyrics of Ireland. Embracing Songs of the Affec
tions, Convivial and Comic Songs, Moral, Sentimental and Satirical Songs Patriotic and Military Songs, Historical and Political Songs, and Miscella neous Songs. Edited and annotated by SAMUEL LOVER, author of "Hand Andy," &c. Embellished with numerous illustrations. 12mo, cloth, gilt side and back. Price---$1 50

---

www.ingramcontent.com/pod-product-compliance
Lightning Source LLC
Chambersburg PA
CBHW083920126
4127000008B/1546